Yoga

Mastering the
BASICS

Yoga

Mastering the
BASICS

Sandra Anderson &
Rolf Sovik, Psy.D.

HIMALAYAN INSTITUTE
PRESS
HONESDALE, PENNSYLVANIA

Himalayan Institute Press
RR1 Box 1129
Honesdale, Pennsylvania 18431–9709

9 8 7 6 5 4 3 2 1

Third printing

*Precautions: Many physical problems benefit from the appropriate practice
of yoga, but please check with your healthcare professional and work with
a well-trained teacher if you have serious health problems. This manual is not
intended to replace personal instruction or professional medical advice. The
contraindications listed for some postures are guidelines only. If you have
abnormal blood pressure, a back injury, or any other serious health problem,
or if you have had surgery recently, please consult with your physician before
beginning your practice.*

Creative direction and design: Jeanette Robertson
Electronic design and production: Julia A. Valenza
Anatomical illustrations: Roger Hill
Computer illustrations: Lucia Lozano
Photography: Jim Filipski, Guy Cali Associates
Models: Ragani Buegel, Luke Ketterhagen, and Bill Boos
Photo, page XII: Nadene Malo
Photo, page 196: Robert Franz / Masterfile
Photo, pages 10, 50, 199: Photodisc, Inc.
Photo, page 218: Anne Arden McDonald / Graphistock
Duotones: C$_2$ media, Inc.

Library of Congress Cataloging-in-Publication Data

Anderson, Sandra.
    Yoga : mastering the basics / Sandra Anderson and Rolf Sovik.
        p. cm.
    Includes index.
    ISBN 0-89389-155-X (pbk. : alk. paper)
     1. Yoga, Hatha. I. Sovik, Rolf. II. Title.

RA781.7 .A488 2000
613.7'046--dc21   99-053823

TO SRI SWAMI RAMA

PRAYERS

GURU BRAHMA

OM Gurur-brahma	OM the Creator is guru
Gurur-vishnur	The Sustainer is guru
Gurur-devo maheshvarah	The Lord of Dissolution is guru
Guruh sakshat param brahma	The supreme Brahman is truly guru
Tasmai shri gurave namah	To that most venerable guru, homage

ASATO MA

Asato ma sad gamaya	Lead me from the unreal to the real
Tamaso ma jyotir gamaya	Lead me from darkness to light
Mrityor ma amritam gamaya	Lead me from mortality to immortality
OM shantih shantih shantih	OM Peace Peace Peace

TEACHER/STUDENT PRAYER

OM saha navavatu	O Lord, may we be protected
Saha nau bhunaktu	May we be nourished and grow in our study
Saha viryam karavavahai	May we create vitality among one another
Tejasvi navadhitamastu	May our study be filled with radiance and energy
Ma vidvishavahai	May there be no enmity among us
OM shantih shantih shantih	OM Peace Peace Peace

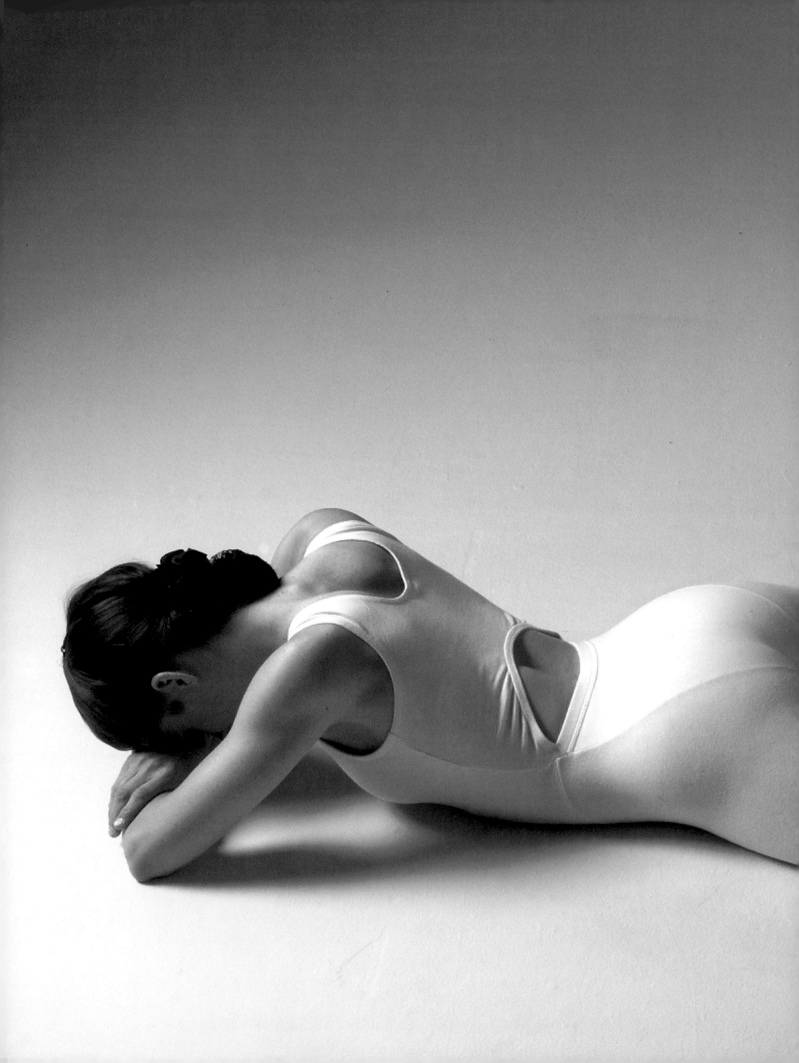

CONTENTS

ACKNOWLEDGMENTS

We are fortunate to have had the help of many friends and colleagues while we prepared this book, and we offer our most sincere thanks to each of them. We are especially grateful to Anne Craig, who handled the complicated editorial demands of this work with grace and an attentive inner ear from start to finish. Similarly, we are most grateful for the thoughtful design work of Jeanette Robertson, whose sensitivity to the aims of the text has greatly enhanced it.

Ragani Buegel, Luke Ketterhagen, and Bill Boos modeled the postures. Sheila Caffrey, Janice Weinstein, and students of the Himalayan Institute in Buffalo, New York, helped review the text in the asana chapters. David Coulter advised us on matters of anatomy. Roger Hill and Lucia Lozano gave great care to the illustrations.

The suggestions and determination of Deborah Willoughby, a devoted yoga student and president of the Himalayan International Institute, have been invaluable in bringing the manuscript to completion. Mary Gail Sovik, co-director of the Himalayan Institute in Buffalo, was an ever-present support whose comments on the developing manuscript, patience through long working hours, and delicious vegetarian cooking kept the fires burning.

Finally, we are deeply indebted to the many teachers from whom we have received inspiration and guidance along the way. In particular we thank the spiritual head of the Himalayan International Institute, Pandit Rajmani Tigunait, for his unfailing encouragement and support.

ABOUT THIS BOOK

In the early stages of practice most yoga students focus on postures, breathing, relaxation, and meditation—combining them into one or two daily sessions of anywhere from 15 to 90 minutes. This is an admirable goal and it is the main theme of this book. But there is much more to yoga, and we have also tried to develop the story further—from philosophy to its application in daily life. Along the way we explore each of the basic components of practice in considerable detail, showing how you can improve your health and sense of inner well-being step by step.

We begin with a chapter called "The Spirit of Yoga" because we think you will want to know about the message behind the practice. An inspiration to students for over four thousand years, yoga philosophy is optimistic and practical. As a companion to the disciplines described in this book, you will find that it deepens both the joy and the mystery of life. If you are looking for stretches and postures, you'll find them in chapters 3, 5, and 6. These chapters include essentially all the poses a beginning student might expect to encounter. Chapter 6 will help you work with problem areas in your body and customize a personal practice.

Breath training, pranayama, relaxation, and meditation are covered in separate chapters. By presenting them in depth it is our hope that a full picture of yoga will begin to emerge—one that unveils its therapeutic potential, as well as the breadth of knowledge it offers for those seeking greater self-awareness.

Breath awareness is so essential to yoga practice it has been said that without it there is no yoga. The essentials are laid out in chapters 4 and 7. If you are troubled by chronic nasal congestion, however, you may want to immediately consider the nasal cleansing described in chapter 7. Relaxation and meditation are treated as an integrated practice that has been explained step by step in chapters 8 and 9. And finally, the experience of yoga in daily life forms the theme of chapter 10. For many, this is what makes yoga come alive—the challenge to continue working on ourselves as an everyday matter.

As authors, we cannot take credit for any of the techniques found here. They belong to a long tradition of teachers and students, and we have tried to pass them along as they are presented within the tradition itself, without personal interpretation. Nonetheless, in yoga personal experience is always the ultimate arbiter and guide—we have learned yoga by doing yoga. It has been a joyful and deeply rewarding experience of self-discovery, self-healing, and self-transformation. We wish the same for you.

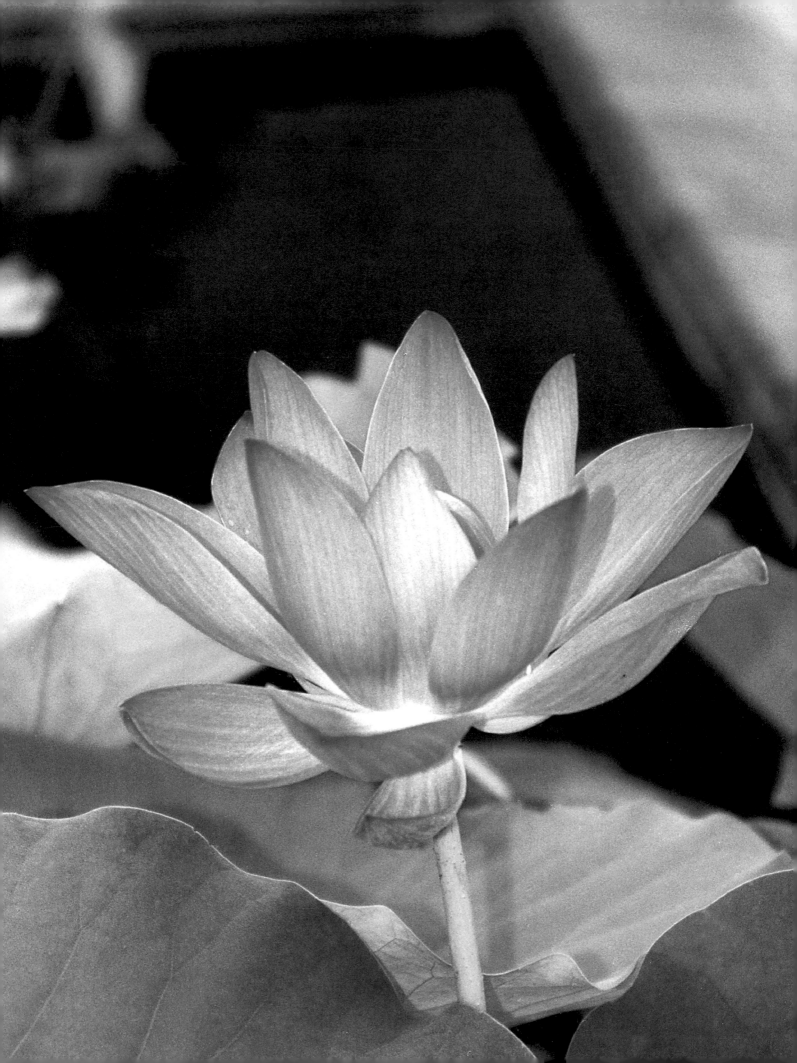

CHAPTER ONE

THE SPIRIT OF YOGA

To know the truth we have to deepen ourselves,
and not merely widen the surface.

———— *Sarvepalli Radhakrishnan*

A N old and revered teacher was working in his garden one day when he was approached by a student who had traveled a considerable distance to see him. Drawing near, the student lowered herself to the ground and sat quietly for a moment. Then, without further hesitation, she asked about the way to enlightenment. The teacher's reply was acted out in the garden dirt. "Pull it up from here," he said, digging beneath an onion plant and uprooting it from the earth. Then, placing the bulb into a hole he had prepared nearby, he added,

"and plant it over here." It is said that the student was enlightened immediately.

Like many enigmatic stories about enlightenment, this one makes good telling, but it is puzzling and a bit difficult to digest. What is particularly challenging is to make the connection between the real-world motives that lead us to yoga and the other-worldly questing for enlightenment found in this story. As new students, we most often turn toward yoga because we are losing our agility, because we need more quiet in our lives, because our health is imbalanced, because we have lost our sense of direction, or because we crave relief from the strain and stress of modern life. Frequently, as new students, we have only a vague idea of what the techniques of yoga are about. We have simply heard that yoga trains the body and mind in a holistic way—and that is appealing enough.

But interestingly, there is a relationship between the metaphor of transplanting onions and the commonsense problems that lead us to begin the study of yoga in the first place. In practice, yoga approaches the job of restoring health and harmony in two ways: by removing obstacles that block our path, and by revealing the unshakable presence of peace, awareness, and joy within. Digging up the onion is the equivalent of rooting out old tensions and pains—detaching from obstacles that make it difficult to learn and to grow. Replanting the onion is a matter of learning to identify with and live in more fertile, inner soil.

Most of us would like to become more flexible, to feel more relaxed, or to manage the chatter of the mind more successfully. But to make these changes we will need a map of the journey. That is the purpose of this first chapter: to provide a brief overview of some of the major philosophical themes of yoga.

DIRECT KNOWLEDGE

Sages of the yoga tradition frequently remind us that each of us is a citizen of two worlds. Each of us dwells simultaneously, they say, in an inner world—a world of thoughts, emotions, and sensations—and an outer world, a universe with which we interact. Our success as human beings depends upon the ability to live skillfully in both worlds. To accomplish this we need a method that will help us to develop self-awareness and at the same time show us how to create harmony in our relationships with the outer world.

It is possible to learn much about life from books and the words of others, but yogis tell us that direct experience provides knowledge of a different and more significant kind. To make this point, a zany story is told about a

mystic who lived his daily life in a city, but whose consciousness was absorbed in self-realization. One day he went to a bank to cash a check. When the teller explained that he must provide two forms of identification, he reached into his wallet and took out a credit card, which he showed to the teller. The teller thanked him and said that just one more proof of identification would be needed. Reaching into his wallet again, the mystic took out a small mirror, looked carefully into it, and proclaimed, "Yes, it's me!"

This story illustrates in an odd way that knowledge acquired from direct experience is altogether different from other kinds of knowledge. When we depend on indirect information about ourselves, it is like relying on the mystic's credit card: the information may be valid, but it cannot show us who we really are. Yoga practices are like the mirror: they allow us to examine ourselves and the source of life directly. They provide firsthand experiential knowledge that is disarmingly revealing and satisfying.

At the heart of yoga is the message that every human being is, by nature, balanced and whole, and that this balanced inner self cannot be permanently destroyed or damaged. It is our inherent nature. Yoga is a method for increasing awareness of this inner self. In the process, each level of personality is given attention because when the body and mind are healthy and when personal conflicts have been resolved, the mind is freed for deeper concentration and reflection.

When such a method is followed systematically it is of profound importance in our lives. Outwardly, it permits us to act in conformity with our needs, our intentions, and the values we hold most dear. Inwardly, we learn to strengthen the body, relax and balance the nervous system, and bring peace and one-pointed concentration to the mind. In the end, yoga is said to lead to the highest goal of life: the direct realization of our own true nature.

THE EIGHT LIMBS OF YOGA

Yoga has been practiced in India for more than forty centuries. But it was not until two thousand years ago that the sage Patanjali codified many already existing practices into a unified text known as the *Yoga Sutras*. Written in the Sanskrit language, this work is a series of terse sentences that convey only the most essential ideas of yoga theory and practice, and so subsequent master teachers have needed to explain these brief aphorisms. Together, Patanjali and his commentators have created a system that can be used to guide students at every level.

The sage Patanjali presented the practices of yoga in the form of eight divisions, or limbs *(ashtanga yoga)*. These eight limbs have become known as *raja* yoga, the "royal" path, because they lead to the complete realization of one's inner nature. The first five limbs are termed the "external" limbs of yoga—practices associated with one's relationships in the world, and with one's body, energy, and senses. Concentration, meditation, and the ultimate goal, *samadhi*, form the second division of the eight limbs and are known as the internal or mental limbs of practice. Although the external rungs of raja yoga form the preliminary steps that strengthen the body and mind, and lead to the practices of meditation, students are not expected to perfect them before proceeding onward. Learning yoga is an organic process, and the various practices mutually clarify and support one another until one-pointed concentration can be achieved.

Surprisingly, the identification of yoga with the many asanas (the stretches and postures commonly illustrated in yoga manuals) is a relatively recent development. In earlier times yoga was primarily associated with contemplative and meditative practices; it was not until roughly a thousand years ago that asanas were widely incorporated into yoga in conjunction with other practices that had been developed to awaken and channel energy. These highly refined techniques, assembled under the name "hatha yoga," not only improved physical and mental health, they also led directly to the spiritual heights of Patanjali's raja yoga as well.

A curious story is told about the origins of modern asana practice. It is said that a fish who happened to be swimming by the seashore one day overheard one of

The 8 Limbs of Raja (Ashtanga) Yoga

Yama	1.	Five Restraints
ahimsa		*non-harming*
satya		*truthfulness*
asteya		*non-stealing*
brahmacharya		*moderation of the senses*
aparigraha		*non-possessiveness*
Niyama	2.	Five Observances
shaucha		*purity*
santosha		*contentment*
tapas		*self-discipline*
svadhyaya		*self-study*
Ishvara pranidhana		*self surrender*
Asana	3.	Posture
Pranayama	4.	Control and Expansion of Energy
Pratyahara	5.	Sense Withdrawal
Dharana	6.	Concentration
Dhyana	7.	Meditation
Samadhi	8.	Self-Realization

the divine beings, the Lord of the Yogis, teaching the secrets of yoga practice to his wife, who had inquired how the suffering of humanity might be relieved. Shortly thereafter that fish gave birth to the human sage Matsyendranath ("Lord of the Fishes"), an adept who was equally revered among hatha yogis, among the tantric practitioners in Tibet and Nepal, and among the practitioners of *rasayana* (a tradition devoted to restoring health and longevity). A perfect master of hatha yoga, he conveyed his knowledge to one of his most famous students, Guru Gorakhnath, and through him a tradition of hatha yoga was passed on that continues today.

The term *yoga*, itself, is derived from the short Sanskrit verb root *yuj*, a word that can be translated "to join or to unite." Through yoga it is said that one may gradually be united with something higher, more subtle, more universal, and more profound than we find in everyday consciousness—the pure nature of the self. Through yoga we discover within ourselves what is normally beyond our capacity; we are yoked to our higher nature, whose existence has the capacity to uplift and transform us.

LAYERS WITHIN LAYERS

Yoga is sometimes described as an inward journey, a movement through the human personality toward the center. Here the word *personality* is not used to mean one's temperament or style of interacting with friends. It means more generally the collection of layers that surround the true nature of the self and serve as an everyday identity (the original meaning of the word *persona* is "mask").

It is said that five dimensions of personality, called *koshas* (sheaths or coverings), surround the self. They function, in effect, like shades around a light—shrouding the intensity and vitality of our self-awareness. As yoga practice proceeds, the sages say, each of these layers will eventually become an integrated part of experience. Each will become more transparent, and as that happens we will experience ourselves with more clarity and energy.

The journey through the koshas is the journey of yoga. It involves turning our awareness inward as we gradually relax and focus the whole personality. The process leads to one-pointed concentration, and this is the vehicle that takes us inward.

THE OUTERMOST MASK

The body, the *annamaya kosha*, is the most visible layer of our personality, and it is the one with which most of us identify. It is made up of the food we eat (*anna* means "food" in Sanskrit). Despite its substantial appearance it is in continual flux—taking in nutrients, eliminating wastes, transforming food into energy, and replacing decaying tissues with new ones. Yet in the midst of this ceaseless activity a sense of inner continuity persists.

There are four instinctive drives—the urges for food, sex (sensual pleasure), sleep, and self-preservation—that accompany the birth of the body, and much of life is consumed in satisfying them. These primitive instincts, in coordination with the senses, lead to our experiences of pleasure and pain. And even though these experiences do not need to impede our inner journey, they often do because of our tendency to focus primarily on sensual gratification. In fact, there are those who say that modern civilization virtually encourages an addictive relationship with the body. And addictive habits of living lead to physical imbalance and poor health.

Preventing illness and managing the body skillfully are important aspects of yoga practice. Just as we must not overindulge the body, we must not deprive it, either.

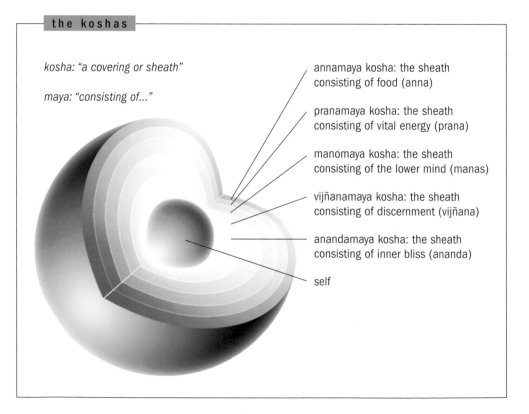

the koshas

kosha: "a covering or sheath"

maya: "consisting of…"

annamaya kosha: the sheath consisting of food (anna)

pranamaya kosha: the sheath consisting of vital energy (prana)

manomaya kosha: the sheath consisting of the lower mind (manas)

vijñanamaya kosha: the sheath consisting of discernment (vijñana)

anandamaya kosha: the sheath consisting of inner bliss (ananda)

self

Yoga is adamantly opposed to extreme asceticism. The message it delivers is that it is important to bring awareness to the body so that we can observe for ourselves how to manage its needs. Periods of asana practice provide concentrated moments for doing this, and they reveal a surprising amount of information about our functioning at a physical level. That is why so much attention is paid to asana practice in this book. But working with diet, sleep patterns, physical relaxation, and cleansing practices is also important in the process of restoring healthy self-awareness. These, together with asanas, are the primary tools for reducing unsound habits of living and preparing the body for the more internal practices to come.

THE ENERGY OF LIFE

The body is formed along the lines of internal energy, called *prana* in Sanskrit. The sheath that consists of prana, the *pranamaya kosha*, is internal to the body and more subtle. So if we wish to know ourselves completely, we will need to acquire experience not only of the body but also of this kosha. The pranamaya kosha is accessed through the breath, and it is through training the breath that our emotional reactions, changes in consciousness (wakefulness and sleep), fluctuations in energy levels, pain, and stress can be moderated. The pranamaya kosha is also associated with more integrated and vibrant experiences of energy that sometimes result from yoga practice.

The study of the breath is a profound science, and one that few of us appreciate. We focus only on the most obvious characteristic of breathing, never suspecting that it may also be a doorway to self-understanding. The quality of everyday breathing influences the quality of life—and breathing can lead us to a state of inner balance if we are willing to study it.

The pranamaya kosha has been repeatedly described as the interface between the body and mind; prana is the force that holds the two together, and thus sustains and regulates life. But prana is not merely a mechanical force—it is a living energy that animates the body and sustains the mind. Every movement and thought is a demonstration of its activity. And by paying attention to the quality of the breath, and to the various states of energy that constitute how we feel, our awareness moves inward and transcends the body. Yoga breathing practices help to regulate and balance prana so that it may be consciously transformed to serve self-awareness.

MEETING THE MIND

Even more subtle than the pranamaya kosha are the next three layers of personality. The most external of these is associated with the conscious mind, the mental screen upon which inner experience is illuminated, called *manas* in Sanskrit. Its sheath, the *manomaya kosha*, provides the self with the capacity for receiving sense impressions, making mental associations, bringing memories into awareness, and coordinating actions. For example, at this very moment, if you choose, you can become aware of your surroundings, of your physical sensations and sense impressions, of the thoughts passing through your mind, or of your relationship to your environment. You can create a chain of thoughts and reflect on it. You can manipulate your body. All these processes are coordinated in the field of the conscious mind.

Our experience is brought to the level of sensation by the annamaya kosha, and to the level of emotions by the pranamaya kosha. At the level of the manomaya kosha it is symbolized in words. But the functioning of the conscious mind is limited. For the most part our perceptions and actions here are automatic and habitual—they are reactions derived from instincts, impulses, and previous experiences. For example, we may plan a vacation and estimate how much money it will cost, but the conscious mind will not be able to determine whether it is wise to carry out our travel plans. For that, we will need to dive to a deeper level of the mind. In other words, at the level of the manomaya kosha we may categorize events in the world clearly, but we will not be able to measure their worth.

INNER WISDOM AND DISCRIMINATION

Traveling inward, the yogis describe two even more subtle layers of the personality. The first, the kosha of wisdom and discrimination, termed the *vijñanamaya kosha*, is the dimension of the self in which the meaning of experience is weighed and recognized. The short Sanskrit verb root *vi-jña*, from which the name of this kosha is derived, means "to discern, to know rightly, to understand." And as our awareness deepens through concentration, we acquire a more clear and accurate vision of ourselves and our relationship to the world, and we act in accordance with it.

Each level of personality draws us closer to our true nature, but at this level the light of the self shines so brightly that from time to time it is not at all uncommon to feel a pull away from the conscious mind toward a deeper and more peaceful inner experience. This level of the self is rarely attained in its full purity, but most meditative states travel the territory between the manomaya and vijñanamaya koshas. Here intuition and discrimination are highly developed, and inner joys replace the distracting excitements of sensual pleasures and emotions.

THE SHEATH OF BLISS

More inward still is the *anandamaya kosha*, named after the Sanskrit word for pure joy or bliss: *ananda.* It is probably the level mystics refer to when their experience has taken them well beyond the distractions of outer life, but not yet to the final destination of the spirit. This is the innermost layer of the personality—not the pure self, but luminous in its light. In rare cases such a state has been attained in a flash by a highly evolved soul, but more often it is attained through pure and one-pointed concentration, nurtured over a long period of practice.

THE CORE OF LIFE

The light of the pure self is said to be beyond the reach of mind and words, and when asked to describe it many sages have chosen silence as their reply. It is better, they say, to let the experience of self-realization unfold without preconception or expectation.

But other sages describe the innermost self as *sat, chit,* and *ananda.* The word *sat* means "true, real, or existent." It carries the idea that the self is beyond all impermanence and can never cease in its existence. *Chit* means "awareness, or consciousness." The self is the subject of experience, never the object. It is an awareness pervading all things. Finally, as we have already seen, *ananda* means "bliss." In the self there is no incompleteness—no lack to create disharmony or pain. The self is full *(purna),* and even when those who know it remain active in the world, they nonetheless dwell in its perfection.

GROWING WHERE WE ARE PLANTED

It is inspiring to understand that the aims of yoga are nothing short of the highest goals of humanity—but we must start where we are planted. For most of us it is equally important to know that it is possible to make practical headway toward happiness in the here and now, in the midst of our own daily lives.

We all know that clustered within the positive experiences of life are those that tax our patience and diminish our optimism. We see evidence of this in our everyday feelings of cynicism, jealousy, sarcasm, and discouragement. To counter these moods Swami Rama, an adept who had considerable influence in the West, often said, "Cheerfulness is the best medicine," and he frequently told this story to illustrate a constructive approach toward "negative karma."

A certain English cleric, a man with scientific interests, decided that he really must consult with Charles Darwin and T. H. Huxley—the foremost champions of the theory of evolution—who had, unfortunately, been dead for decades. Undeterred, the cleric received permission to visit heaven, but after a thorough check St. Peter was not able to find the names of these two great men on the list of the heavenly enrolled. Reluctantly he sent the cleric down the road to visit "the other place." When he got there the cleric was surprised to discover that hell had an even more impressive gate than the pearly gates of heaven—this one was covered with jewels and precious stones. When he rang the bell and the doors were opened, they revealed a grassy expanse with fountains, flowers, and trees. Deer wandered through the park, and birds sang sweetly. Puzzled, the cleric asked if Darwin and Huxley were there. The gatekeeper pointed out the two. "They're the ones planting flowers over by the base of the wading pool," he said. "You're welcome to pay them a visit."

But before setting out, the cleric made an offhand comment to the gatekeeper. "You know," he said, "where I come from on Earth, hell has a reputation for being quite awful—unbearably hot, ugly, and painful, in fact."

"Oh yes," said the gatekeeper. "Well, you should have seen the place before Darwin and Huxley arrived!"

This story is worth pondering. It contains the essence of cheerfulness and the seed for a dynamic shift in attitude about our life here on Earth.

THE PATHS
OF YOGA

There are many paths for you to follow on your inward journey—one for every type of personality. But the task of sorting them out can be confusing. Contemporary teachers have invented new names and reinterpreted old ones to distinguish their particular styles from one another, and as a result it may seem as if modern yoga schools are mutually exclusive. If you are familiar with the main paths of classic yoga, however, it will be easy to determine the goals of

contemporary schools. And the style of yoga you choose to focus on will stabilize as your interests and needs solidify and as you meet teachers who can provide reliable guidance.

A classic text of ancient India, the *Bhagavad Gita*, describes four paths of yoga, but as you think about them remember that no yoga path is entirely separate from the others. Differences among them have developed out of differences in individual temperament. The final goal remains the same.

The four paths described in the *Gita* have been likened to the body of a bird in flight.

1 ASHTANGA YOGA

The eight limbs of raja yoga are sometimes called the "yoga of practice." They are compared to the head of the bird. They provide the disciplines, guidance, organization, and vision that are necessary for flight, and these are shared in common among all the paths of yoga. The other three paths, which are associated

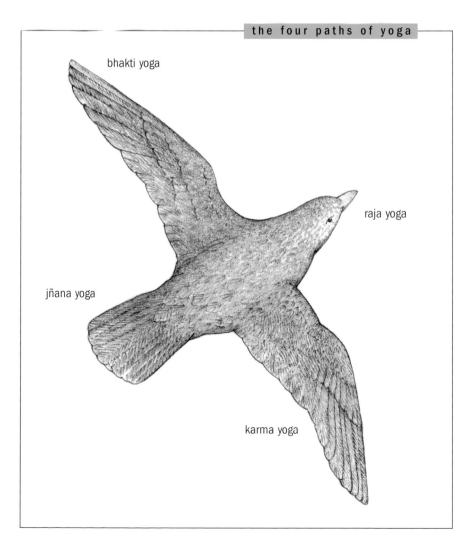

the four paths of yoga

bhakti yoga

raja yoga

jñana yoga

karma yoga

with the wings and tail of the bird, are sometimes called the "yogas of life" because they use one's natural tendencies as a means for self-realization, and illustrate how yoga can be achieved in the midst of ordinary activities.

2   KARMA YOGA

Karma yoga consists of performing actions without expectation or selfish attachment. Karma yoga is especially suited for those who are action-oriented; it brings a sense of inner balance in the midst of activity. Whether it be painting the kids' bedroom, helping out at the charity marathon, or simply performing one's daily duties, it is karma yoga as long as the action is performed skillfully and without selfish regard for the outcome of the action. Such actions propel life forward productively. This is equally true for the benefactor who anonymously donates millions of dollars to charity, for the stagehand who voluntarily labors behind the scenes to make the community theater a success, and for the family member who cheerfully does the dishes even when it is not his turn. The key to karma yoga is the selflessness that motivates the action. Regarding this path, the *Bhagavad Gita* says:

Fixed in yoga, perform your actions, abandoning attachment and remaining equal in success and failure; for yoga is equanimity, it is said. (2:48)

3   BHAKTI YOGA

The bird's other wing is the path of devotion, or bhakti yoga (from the Sanskrit *bhaj*, "to turn or resort to; to adore or to love"). Musicians, artists, poets, and those whose joy lies in the refinement of sentiment often find themselves attracted to this path. But again, it is wise not to define bhakti yoga too narrowly. It is not just for artists. The practice of every yoga student thrives if there is some measure of love and appreciation for the teachings. Without an element of bhakti any practice becomes dry.

The path of bhakti is characterized not only by love, but by faith and surrender as well. While yoga is not a religion, it does not ignore the fact that human hearts need an object of affection just as human minds need an object of concentration. The goals of yoga are worthy of reverence and devotion, and such devotion, itself, can lead to self-realization. That is the message here. It is expressed in many verses in the *Gita*. The following ones are spoken by Krishna, an embodiment of the yogic ideal which is within all of us:

Because of your faith I shall tell you what is most secret—knowledge combined with experience—and having known it you will be released from every impurity. (9:1)

4   JÑANA YOGA

Finally, there are some whose joy and sense of fulfillment is found in the study of philosophy, the careful analysis of life, and the development of dispassion regarding worldly activities. Such persons are inclined to the path of jñana yoga, a path that emphasizes awareness and discrimination. Jñana yoga is likened to the tail of the bird, since it is the tail, the rudder, that gives direction in flight.

The path of jñana yoga is about more than mere intellect, however. Through this path we develop the ability to see our mind and personality dispassionately, witnessing passions and distractions yet remaining above them. Regarding one who practices jñana yoga, the *Gita* says:

One who sits dispassionately, unmoved by changing conditions, thinking "It is only the play of nature," standing firm and unwavering; regarding pain and pleasure alike, dwelling in the Self . . . such a one is said to have risen above . . . (14:23–25)

Thus the power to move through life is propelled by the wings of bhakti and karma yoga. One's orientation in life is adjusted by the tail feathers of jñana yoga. And the practices of raja yoga provide one with the experience to guide life's flight wisely.

Other Paths of Yoga

There are other important paths in yoga, each associated with a particular style and approach. They are often thought to be distinct, but they are thoroughly integrated with one another in both practice and philosophy. They include:

▶ **Mantra Yoga**
A path of self-realization that uses various vocal sounds and words as a means of transcendental guidance and support. Certain mantras are used almost exclusively for meditation, while others function as prayers, accompaniments to rituals, or tools for contemplation. Mantra practice is commonly a part of raja yoga.

▶ **Kundalini Yoga**
A path associated with the awakening and gradual assimilation of the dormant energy of individual consciousness. On this path the various centers of consciousness that lie along the spinal axis, the chakras, are described. The practices of hatha yoga are closely related to the theory and practice of kundalini yoga.

▶ **Tantra Yoga**
A path in which the relationship between individual consciousness and the universe is systematically explored, and the knowledge is used for self-realization. Tantra yoga is characterized by disciplines which combine mantra, visualization, external and internal ritual, and many aspects of ashtanga yoga. Its practice requires a precise technique and extensive knowledge of many aspects of yoga.

THE FLIGHT INTO SILENCE

As you might have gathered by now, there is far greater scope to yoga than can be covered in this brief chapter. And as your discovery is just beginning, to weigh it down with more concepts would only needlessly postpone your enjoyment. In fact, concepts about yoga, no matter how concisely they are summarized, soon begin to reflect the limitations of words and language and become an obstacle to experiencing what yoga offers.

The deep stream of inner life cannot be described. Throughout the history of the yoga tradition this fact has led teachers and students alike to take periodic refuge in a flight from spoken words and labored concepts— into silence. Silence makes it possible to explore the parts of ourselves that otherwise pass unacknowledged and unobserved. With this in mind, yoga classes are most often taught without a musical backdrop, instructions are carefully presented but kept to a minimum, and attention is shepherded to the quiet activity of self-observation.

Systematic experiences of silence, such as those in meditation, are among the most gratifying aspects of yoga study. In silence there is room for emotion and thought to evolve. Doorways open to self-understanding, and self-acceptance can blossom. Silence makes it possible to calm our social expectations and listen to the necessities of our own life. And the confidence developed during periods of silence can translate into a ready confidence at other times as well.

But by now you must be eager to begin your practice. The next chapter provides the guidelines you will need to practice safely and effectively. Take time to review them, and then don't hesitate to begin.

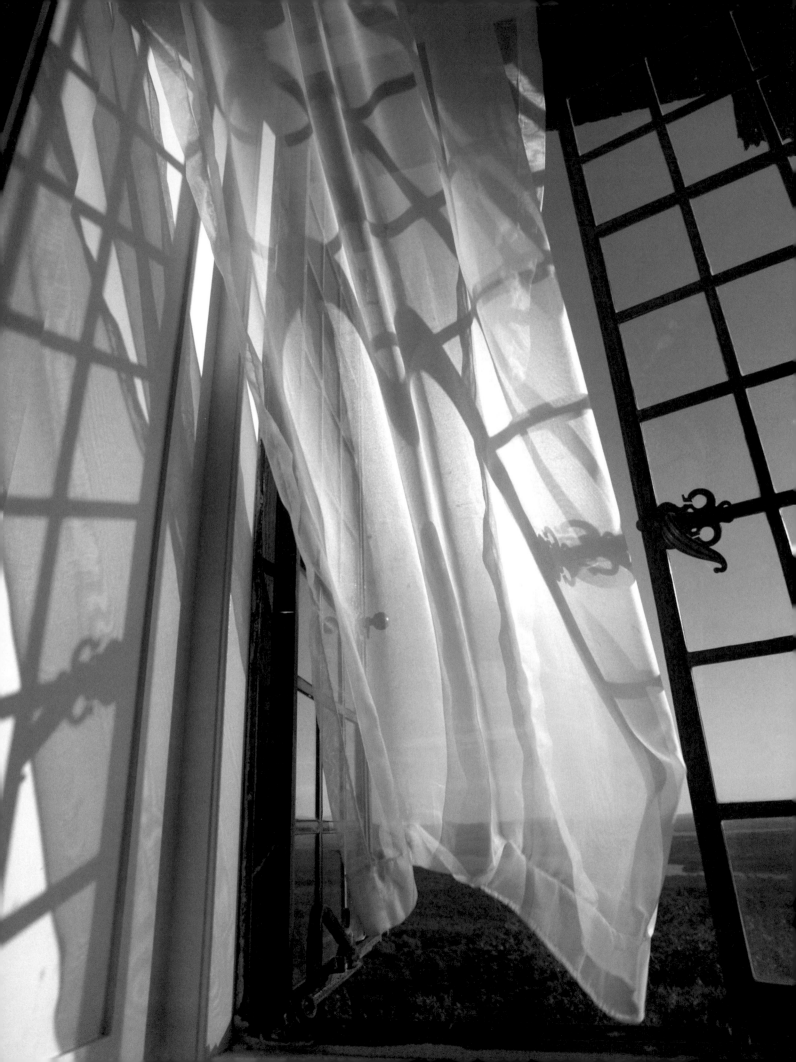

GETTING STARTED

I F you have never practiced yoga before, you are about to encounter yourself in a fresh and uplifting way. All the disciplines of yoga are intended for one purpose: to awaken in you a renewed sense of balance and harmony that will gradually reintroduce you to yourself. A few guidelines will help you begin—to a large extent they are answers to questions you may have already framed in your mind, or soon will once you have started your practice.

For example, you will want to know what kind of space is most suitable for practice; what style of clothing to wear; what are the best moments in the day for practice; and how much time to set aside for it. Other, more nebulous queries may have passed through your mind as well: How will you know if you are performing the exercises correctly? What is supposed to happen as the sequence of stretches and postures progresses? How long will it take to notice progress? The purpose of this chapter is to set the stage for you to begin.

In the beginning, naturally, our focus is on learning a repertoire of stretches and postures. We need to attend to the basics of placing and aligning the body, and to work through muscular weaknesses and tensions that make some postures difficult or inaccessible. To this end, a few words on stretching muscles are in order.

STRETCHING

Stretching feels good. It is easy to lose sight of that when our daily routine keeps us sitting too long, when our neck and shoulders are crying out for a massage, and when we are growing sleepier by the minute. Stretching awakens the body. Within a few minutes muscles feel warm, tightness loosens its grip, and a sudden surge of energy gives the impression that weary brain cells have come alive again. Stretching is invigorating—and that is the start of the inner dance called yoga.

Stretching also makes us more flexible—a term that may seem familiar but is difficult to define. Technically, flexibility is the ease and range of motion at a joint. But we all experience some limitations in our movements, and we all have joints that move normally as well. Individual differences are the rule. For example, forward bending may be a strong point for one person, while for another it is difficult. The same person who bends forward with ease may find that twisting or backward bending presents problems. In yoga, we start where we are—not where our expectations tell us to be. And whenever we discover tension, whether subtle or obvious, it presents an opportunity for freeing blocked energy and rigidity.

What creates resistance to flexibility? This is an important question. Some joint resistance is structural and cannot be changed, but most resistance varies from day to day—and over a lifetime. The three main areas

that concern us, as yoga students, are tightness in muscles and connective tissue, habits of posture and movement that unconsciously reinforce joint restrictions, and mental states that lead to physical tension. If we are to bring about change through yoga, we must work with each of these.

OVERCOMING RESISTANCE

When muscles are stretched, they give us internal feedback because stretch receptors, found in the belly of muscles, automatically stop us from stretching too far or too fast. Overburdened stretch receptors signal a muscle to resist, and this prevents successful stretching. That is why yoga stretches are performed slowly and include ample periods of relaxed holding. That way stretch receptors can be re-educated and a new level of flexibility achieved.

Sheaths of connective tissue, called fascia, weave through and around muscles, and rigidity in this fascia also creates resistance to stretching—the web of tissue holding the muscles becomes increasingly less pliable. Yoga stretches provide the perfect tool for restoring natural elasticity to these connective fibers and making them more supple.

Another source of muscle tension is remaining in one position too long. In the not too distant past the entire human race spent a good deal of time walking; a purely sedentary life was rare. But within the past hundred years this has changed dramatically. Now it is possible to go through life with virtually no vigorous movement and with long periods of sitting, and the result is increased muscle rigidity and tension. The variety of movements incorporated into a balanced sequence of yoga stretches and postures reverses this trend—the entire body receives the benefits of regular movement, and mobility is improved.

A third reason for muscle tension is that as flexibility declines it is natural for us to accommodate joint restrictions by changing the way we use our body. For example, rather than actually turning to look behind us as we back the car, we begin to rely on mirrors. This and similar habits reinforce the tension we were already feeling, creating a vicious circle. We need new options—and the wide range of stretches available in yoga provides exactly that. The postures allow us to recover movements that have been sacrificed to tension, and to reacquaint ourselves with the pleasure of unrestricted movement.

Finally, mental states can affect flexibility. Most of us know what it is like to feel tight and physically restless under emotional stress. And when these conditions become chronic they reduce flexibility in increasingly visible ways: poor posture, fatigue, and obvious limitations in movement. Chronic tension may also result in headaches or more serious nerve pain.

Physical stretching alone may not be entirely successful in relieving stress, so we must learn to work with ourselves at every level. But asana practice sessions do help by getting at embedded muscle tension, and they provide other powerful tools (such as relaxed breathing and a non-judgmental approach to ourselves) that can actively reduce nervous system strain as well. Then we can stretch "from the inside out."

STRATEGIES FOR PRACTICE

There are a number of ways to stretch. One that most of us are familiar with from gym class stretches muscles rapidly by bouncing in and out of fixed positions. This is called ballistic stretching because it suddenly hurls (Latin *ballista:* "to throw") a portion of the body into a stretch. The movement is often unconscious—our mind can be far away while the body goes through its routine of bouncing and moving.

Most of us have experienced the stiffness that follows this kind of stretching, and because stiffness results from micro tearing in the fibers of muscles, injury can easily result. Stiffness is usually not a sign of severe damage, however, and by the second day after stretching it will generally improve. But it makes stretching uncomfortable and prohibits us from progressing smoothly.

Yoga postures, on the other hand, are usually done slowly, with periods of holding at the point of the stretch. Or if the stretch involves repetitive movement,

the repetition itself allows for a period of observation. Whether slow and deliberate with periods of holding the stretches, or repetitive and involving naturally paced movement, yoga stretches are always accompanied by awareness of one's whole body.

THE INNER OBSERVER

The essence of yoga is skillful self-observation, and when you are performing a yoga stretch or posture your inner observer needs to be awake. You may find that the pose you are performing challenges muscles you had not expected to be affected, or that it summons your balance skills, but not your flexibility. You may notice that your breathing is disturbed by a certain posture and that the pull to come out of it is more closely related to anxiety than to muscle fatigue. You may even discover that moving your body requires far less effort than you had imagined it would and that stretching introduces you to an ease of movement you had not anticipated. Observing your body, breath, and mind during the stretch is the only way to learn the lessons each stretch can provide.

Stretching will also lead you to make further observations—about your health, the way you relate to your body, your stress levels and coping skills, your mental habits and reaction patterns, and your ability to relax and concentrate. And because many of us can be fierce critics of ourselves, it is helpful from the outset to remember that this is not a competitive or fault-finding process. Your task in yoga is to see yourself positively, and to perform the stretches and postures with care.

BODY, BREATH, AND MIND

The key to bringing awareness to a yoga posture is to observe what is going on inside it. Then with practice you will learn to make adjustments so that the flow of energy you experience internally establishes the body in the most balanced alignment possible. Your goal is to develop ease and stability. Imposing an idealized notion of what a posture should look like can create tension or even injury, so stay present with the physical sensations arising inside you. Be aware of inner boundaries. At the same time, explore the edges of your awareness, sensing what you might be missing when your attention wanders, or conversely, when you focus too intently.

Breath awareness is an important way to maintain this "soft" focus; being conscious of the breath allows you to "listen" to the impression that is being made by the posture as a whole. It's not unlike listening to a symphony orchestra: from time to time you shift your awareness to the violins, the French horns, or the timpani, but you do that within the context of the sound of the entire orchestra. Similarly, awareness of the breath allows you to observe delicate physical sensations, patterns of internal energy, and even passing thoughts, yet remain aware of the internal unity of the pose.

When approached in this way, each stretch or yoga posture becomes a vehicle for self-awareness, and its effects are magnified by actively collaborating with it rather than resisting its challenges. You will learn to perform the pose correctly—the methods for entering, holding, and leaving it. You will be able to identify the range of effects each posture has on the body, breath, and mind, and reap the benefits of practice. Does the pose require strength? Then by slowly increasing your holding time you will develop a stronger body. Does the pose require balance? Then regular practice will improve your concentration. Are you anxious in the pose? Then relaxed breath awareness will help you uncover the source of your tension and transform your perception of the pose as well as your self-confidence.

In the process you will find that learning to respond to each posture and stretch from the inside out is a gratifying challenge. Your knowledge of your body will grow; you will feel more coordinated in your movements; your posture will improve; your circulation will improve and wastes will be eliminated from your body more efficiently; your breathing will deepen; and overall, your efforts will contribute to a positive self-image. The postures will then begin to flow naturally, each arising out of your own awareness of what needs to be done to bring yourself into mental, physical, and spiritual harmony.

GUIDELINES FOR PRACTICE

Here are some answers to the most commonly asked questions about yoga. They are guidelines, not rules, and after reading them through you'll be ready to start on the sequence of stretches and postures in the next chapter.

What is the best environment for practice?

Practice in a clean, quiet, well-ventilated, and peaceful space with a firm carpet or other non-skid surface. Avoid temperature extremes, direct sun, and drafts.

Are special clothes necessary?

Wear non-binding clothes such as a tee shirt and sweatpants, tights, or shorts; take off your shoes and socks. Natural fabrics allow the skin to breathe. If you can do without your glasses, take them off during your practice period.

What about special equipment?

Yoga requires refreshingly little in the way of extra equipment, although numerous props and aids for practice are available. You will need a thin cushion (for relaxation and meditation) and a blanket or shawl to cover your body on cold days. You may also want to own a canvas strap (to help with postures that are "just out of reach"); a non-skid mat (to keep the footing solid); and an eye pillow (to darken daytime light during relaxation).

How do I coordinate practice with meals and digestion?

The postures affect the internal organs, so it is better to wait until they are no longer busy with digestion. Practice on an empty stomach and bladder. You will feel better if the bowels are also empty, and some practices require this. Wait about two hours after a light meal and four hours after a heavy meal.

What is the best time for practice?
How much time is needed?

For practicing yoga postures, early morning and late afternoon (before the evening meal) have traditionally been recommended. Some people also find that a series of light stretches an hour before bedtime is relaxing. You may have a time in your schedule that naturally works well, and if so, then that will be the best time for you.

A minimum of about 15 minutes is needed to complete a short sequence of stretches and a brief relaxation; 30 minutes will provide time for more stretching and a complete relaxation. The two sequences contained in this book require from 45 minutes to an hour, depending upon the pace of the practice and the number of times each pose is repeated.

Regular systematic practice is the most effective. Try to practice at least three times a week. Daily practice is ideal. The time you spend depends on your schedule (see chapter 10). It is better to be regular with a 15-minute session than sporadic with a longer practice. In setting a schedule be kind to yourself and be realistic.

What about illness or recent injury?

Yoga can be an invaluable tool in recovering from illness or injury, but your practice must match the stage of your recovery. Do not practice prematurely or exceed your capacity. Use breathing and relaxation techniques first, then add stretches as your body can tolerate them. Injuries and surgeries require rest before recuperative work begins. Stress-related mental health problems

Some Basic Suggestions

Start each session with a brief relaxation (1–3 minutes), and end with a thorough relaxation.

Breathe evenly through the nose throughout the session. Do not hold the breath.

Keep the eyes soft but open.

Do not strain or force to reach or to hold a position. Let the movements flow from one to the next.

Nurture feelings of lightness, elongation, and strength. In each pose ask yourself how to deepen your experience of it; how to lengthen the spine; how to feel stronger, steadier, and more spacious in the pose. Even curled into a ball you'll want to be aware of the space in the joints of the shoulders and hips, and the length of the back of the neck and spine.

Pay attention. Focus on the sensations in the entire body as you work. Be sensitive and be aware as you experience the postures. Energy follows thought—that is, energy goes where you direct your attention. Be aware not only of where you feel a stretch, but also of how the whole body is responding.

Remain in the present. When thoughts pull you away to other times or places, use the sensations of your body and breath to return to the room and to the work you are doing with yourself.

In general, you should feel good after a pose; better than before. Any discomfort while you are holding the pose should immediately dissipate when the posture releases, leaving a sense of well-being. Except for joint disease, pain in the joints during or after a pose indicates incorrect practice. Likewise, unusual pressure in the eyes, ears, or head is a sign to modify your practice. If you don't feel relaxed and energized after your session, you may be overdoing it.

respond well to yoga. Unlike physical illness or injury, mental health problems can emphasize work with postures (in addition to breathing and relaxation) to help the mind become well-grounded and steady. But yoga is not a substitute for medical care. If a health problem persists, see a qualified medical adviser.

How does menstruation affect practice?

During menstruation avoid inverted poses, overexertion, and pressure or heat in the abdomen. For many women this is a good time to rest, concentrating more on relaxation postures and on breathing and meditation exercises. Others may find relief from the discomfort of menstruation in gentle stretches. Do not overdo.

When will I begin to see progress?

You may feel better from the first session—yoga is that effective. But progress is often one of the most difficult things to evaluate in ourselves. Unexpectedly, however, one day a friend or colleague will remark to you that you seem more calm, or more energetic. Until then you might measure your progress by how you feel when you skip your practice. That "something is missing" feeling means that you have experienced a new benchmark of calmness in your body and mind, and want to get back to it.

What about yoga classes?

Take classes. There is no substitute for a teacher. Find a class that works for you, and attend it. A good class will give you valuable feedback, reinforce your commitment, refresh your practice, add techniques and poses to your repertoire, and perhaps most importantly, it will provide *satsanga*—the company of like-minded people to uplift and inspire you on the yoga path.

A Final Thought

Enjoy your practice! Practice for the joy and satisfaction of the process. One of the cornerstones in the foundation of yoga is non-attachment to the fruits of your actions. So practice for the pleasure of it. On days when the pleasure of it is not immediately apparent (and there will be days like that), find pleasure in the discipline.

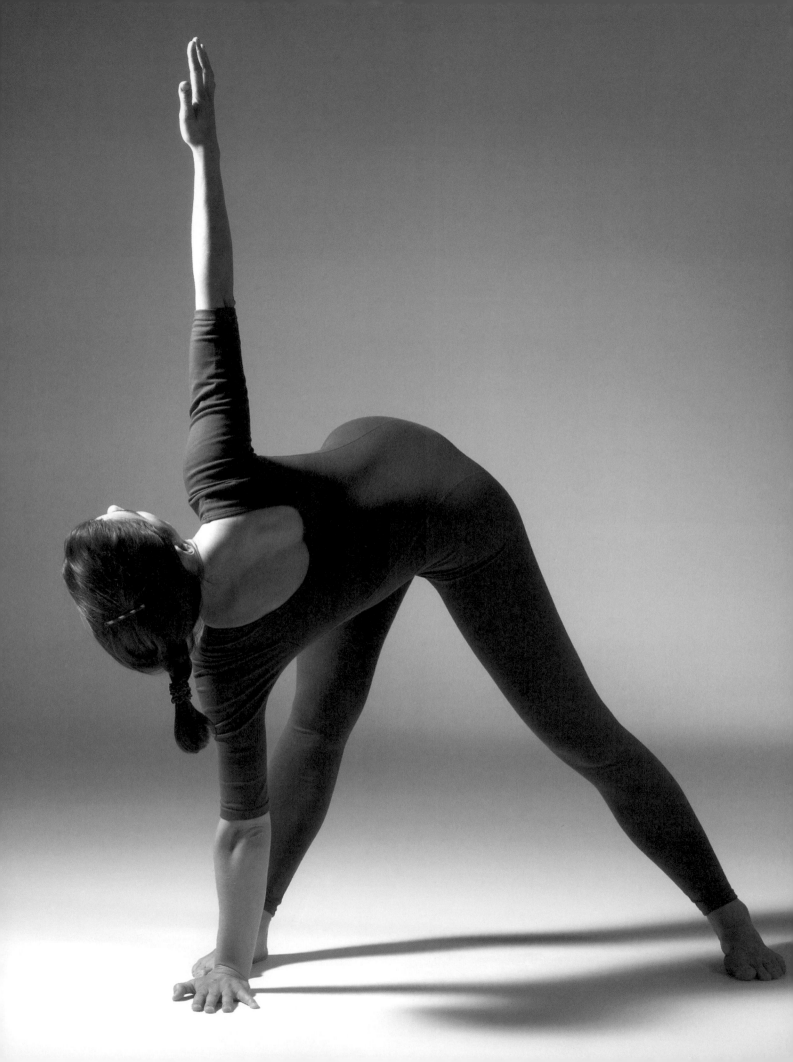

CHAPTER THREE

ASANA SEQUENCE ONE

Hatha yoga is a sheltering retreat for those scorched
by all types of pain. For those engaged in the practice
of every kind of yoga, hatha yoga is like the tortoise
that supports the world.
———— *Hatha Yoga Pradipika*

flexibility, strength, and balance

GIVEN the hectic conditions of modern life, few of us find time to grant our body and mind the care they need to function properly. A simple sequence of yoga asanas, or postures, however, and a few minutes of regular practice can go a long way toward maintaining optimal health. The following progression is designed to tone the whole body, and it will bring about greater flexibility, strength, balance, and coordination, as well as a clearer, more focused mind. It provides a wide range of stretches that, taken together, will move virtually every joint in your body, and as you work your way through the sequence you will learn how to use these stretches most effectively. Review the descriptions and illustrations carefully in order to understand how to perform each stretch accurately. Then the practice itself will become your teacher.

For those who are just beginning hatha yoga or for anyone who wants a gentle rejuvenating practice, this is an ideal sequence. It is comprehensive but does not require the flexibility, strength, or stamina of more difficult practices, and it is an excellent preparation for all yoga asanas. Some of the exercises are good training for specific postures; others stretch or strengthen in general preparation for later work. The complete sequence is pictured at the end of this chapter. When you are comfortable with this sequence you can progress to the more challenging postures in chapter 5.

This sequence can also serve as a maintenance program if you are not interested in advancing in the postures but would like to maintain a healthy body and the capacity to practice other aspects of yoga. The ancient texts, in fact, tell us that hatha yoga is the foundation and support for all other yoga practices. The following sequence of warm-ups and beginning-level poses will provide that foundation.

Crocodile Pose (Makarasana)

Lie face down. Fold your arms, each hand on the opposite elbow, and draw the forearms in so that the chest is slightly off the floor and the forehead rests on the crossed forearms. Keep the legs together, or separate them a comfortable distance with the toes turned either out or in. Close your eyes, and relax the legs, abdomen, shoulders, and face. Turn your attention to the breath. Feel the cleansing flow of the exhalation and the rejuvenating flow of the inhalation. Remain in the pose for about 15 breaths.

▶ Benefits: Establishes deep, relaxed breathing; centers awareness; brings attention into the present.

Crocodile Pose (Makarasana)

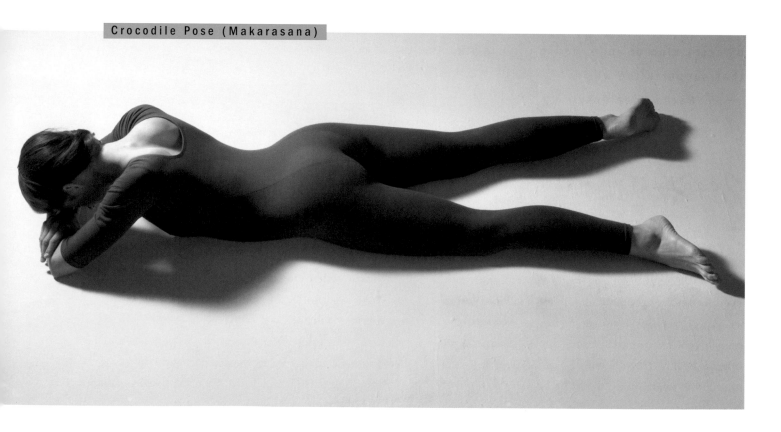

Symmetrical Stretch

Roll onto your back. Bring your feet together and stretch the arms overhead on the floor with the palms facing each other. While keeping the left side relaxed, lengthen the entire right side of the body, stretching both the right arm and the right leg. Then change sides, alternately stretching 5 times on each side. Finally, bring your legs together and stretch up through both arms, broadening the upper back as you simultaneously lengthen both legs. Hold this stretch for 5 breaths. Feel the abdomen rise and fall as you breathe. Then release on an exhalation.

▶ Benefits: Stretches the muscles and connective tissues of the whole body. Prepares for many other yoga postures.

Reclining Side Stretch

Lying on your back with the legs together, interlace the fingers behind the head. Slide your upper body to the right, keeping the upper back, pelvis, and back of the legs flat on the floor. Walk the heels to the right, stretching the entire left side of the body. Keep the ankles and legs together, and don't allow the left hip or shoulder to come off the floor. Take 3–5 breaths and explore the stretch. As you relax you may be able to bend the torso a bit further to the right. Release the stretch and come back to center. Then repeat on the other side.

▶ Benefits: Stretches the side of the torso from the hip to the shoulder; facilitates full, easy breathing.

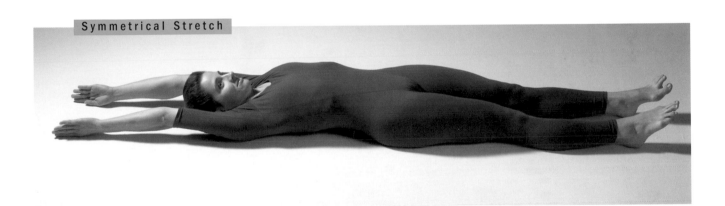

Symmetrical Stretch

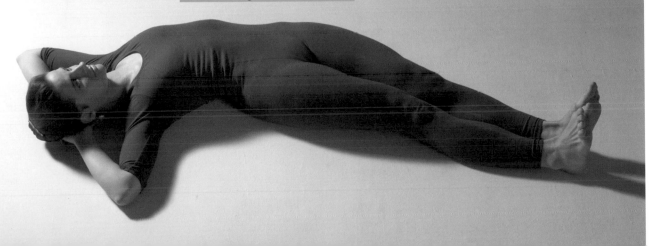

Reclining Side Stretch

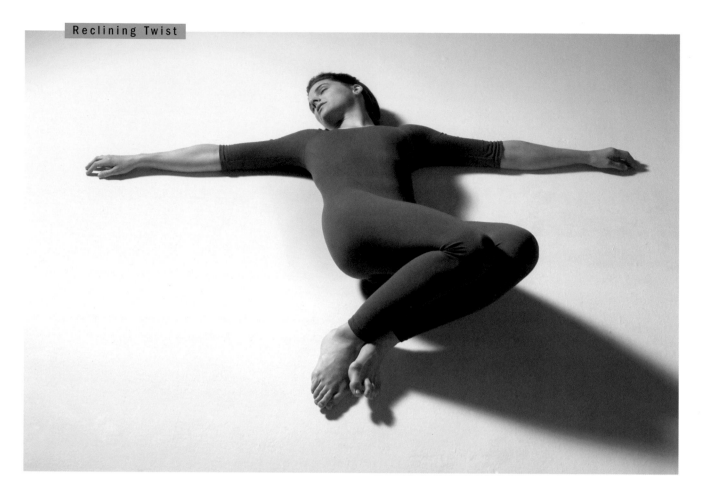

4

Reclining Twist

Lie on your back with the arms out to the sides, palms down. Bend the knees, and place the feet on the floor near the pelvis, hip-width apart. Keeping your feet on the floor, exhale and twist your lower body to the left, lowering the knees gently toward the floor. Inhale and return to the center, then exhale and repeat on the right side. You may also turn the head in the opposite direction from the knees. Repeat 3–5 times on each side. To deepen the twist and strengthen the abdomen, raise the knees toward the chest. Keeping the legs firmly together, twist from side to side as before. Then roll to the left side, and sit up.

▶Benefits: Releases tension from the mid- and lower back; gently twists the spine and abdomen.

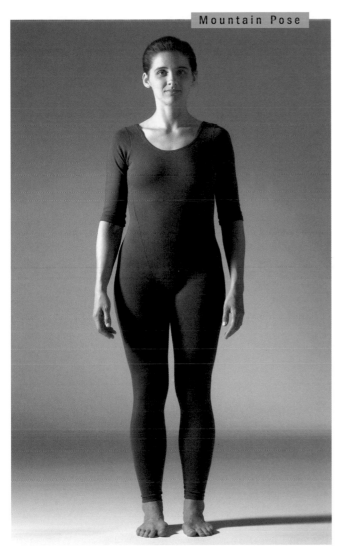

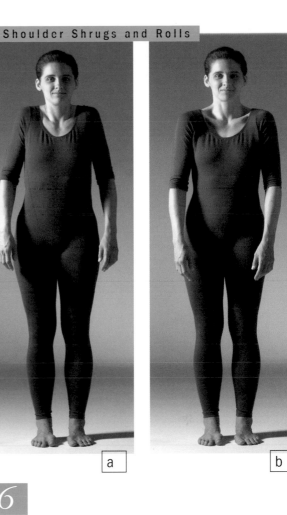

a   b

6

5

Mountain Pose (Tadasana)

Stand with your feet parallel and hip-width apart, toes pointed straight forward. Roll the shoulders up and back and release them so that the arms rest alongside the body. Let your spine be erect and your weight balanced over the arches of the feet. Spread the toes and press down evenly through the soles of the feet as you lift up through the top of the head. Hold for 3–5 breaths.

▶ Benefits: Establishes a neutral, balanced alignment of the body that provides an inner reference for standing and other poses. Brings awareness to posture in daily life.

Shoulder Shrugs and Rolls

a) Inhale and lift both shoulders toward the ears. Exhale and drop the shoulders. Repeat 3 times.

b) Then roll the shoulders, circling them forward, up, back, and down. Inhale as the shoulders lift and roll back, and exhale as they lower and roll forward. After 3–5 rotations, change direction. Strive for full extension in all directions, keeping the arms and hands passive and relaxed.

▶ Benefits: These and the following four exercises help to open, strengthen, and realign the shoulders, thus restoring the full range of movement. They will noticeably improve circulation to the entire upper torso.

Arm Circles

Stand erect with the arms resting at the sides. Lift both arms out to the side and parallel to the floor, palms facing down. Keep the shoulders relaxed. Circle the arms, starting with small movements and gradually increasing the size of the circles until they are as big as possible. Maintaining the full movement, change direction and gradually decrease the size of the circles, returning to the starting position. Then lower the arms.

Vertical Arm Swings

Stand erect with the palms of the hands facing the sides. Make a light fist and swing the arms forward and backward, feeling your chest and shoulders open as the arms swing back. To increase the momentum of the movement, on alternate swings bend the elbows, thrusting them backward. Continue for 20–30 seconds.

Arm Circles

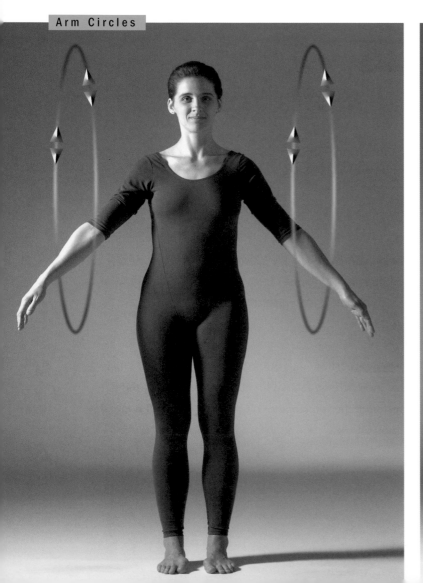

Vertical Arm Swings

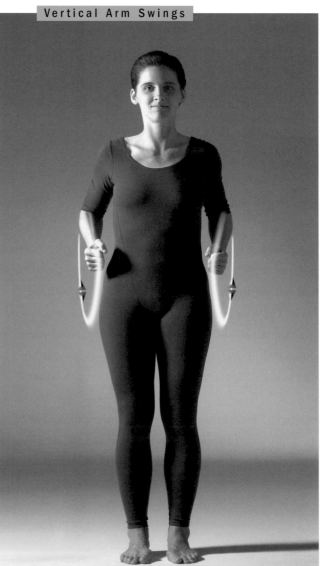

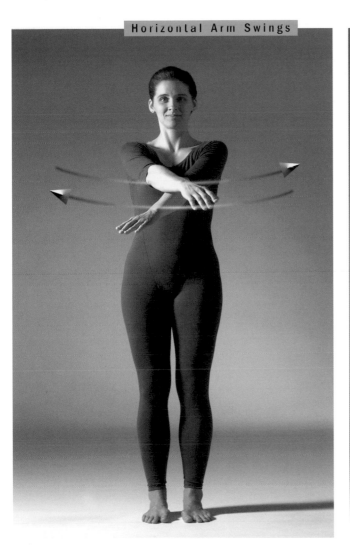

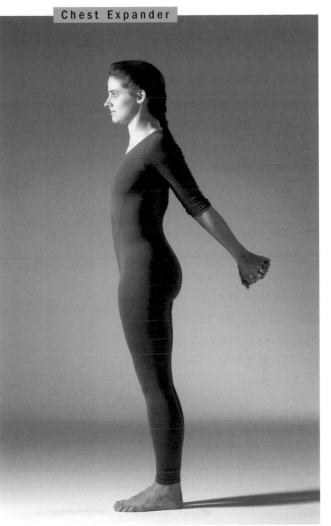

Horizontal Arm Swings

Stand erect, raising your arms out to the sides and parallel
to the floor. Now swing the arms forward and back,
alternating the arm on top as the arms cross in the front.
For full extension, release resistance in the upper chest
as you swing back, drawing the shoulder blades toward
each other. Continue for 20–30 seconds.

Chest Expander

Stand erect and clasp your hands behind you. Draw the
shoulders back and press the shoulder blades toward
each other. If possible bring the palms of the hands
together, and straighten the elbows, lengthening the
arms toward the floor. Hold the stretch and breathe,
opening the chest. To deepen the stretch, lift the arms
away from the back while raising and expanding the
chest. Keep the spine erect, lengthing the neck and
the lower back. Breathe deeply for 3–5 breaths in
each position.

Standing Warm-Up Twist

Stand with the feet slightly more than shoulder-width apart. Form a light fist, and bend your elbows so that the arms are held near the waist. With your head facing forward, twist the torso from side to side at a moderate pace, breathing naturally. To deepen the twist gradually increase the movement of the shoulders and hips, but maintain control and do not overstretch. Breathe evenly throughout. Continue for 30–40 seconds.

▸<u>Benefits</u>: Improves flexibility of the spine and circulation to the torso.

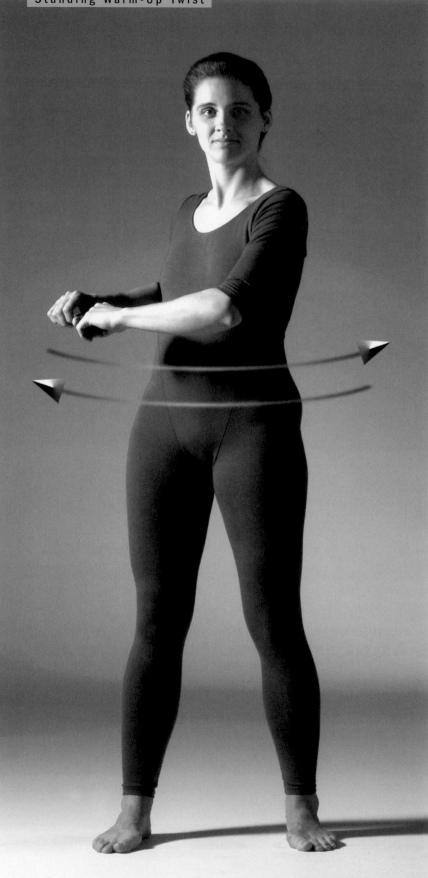

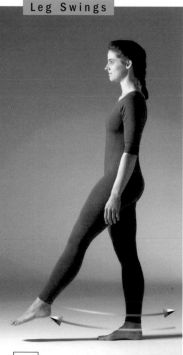

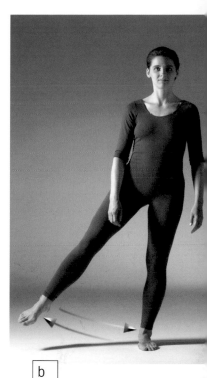

a

b

12

Supported Torso Rotation

Stand with the feet about 2 feet apart. Support your lower back with the palms of your hands, fingers spread and pointing downward. Bend slightly forward to begin, then rotate the hips to the right, then forward, then left, then back, in a circling movement. You might imagine that you are standing in a barrel, swabbing the inside rim with your pelvis. Allow the head and shoulders to shift as needed to balance the pelvis. Rotate 5 times in each direction.

▶Benefits: Improves coordination; limbers the hips, pelvis, and lower back.

13

Leg Swings

a) Stand in the mountain pose with feet together. Keeping both knees straight, swing one leg straight forward, and then straight back. Repeat 10 times. Keep the torso and pelvis upright and steady.

b) Next swing the leg straight out to the side 5–10 times. Keep the toes facing forward and the pelvis stable, as before.

Repeat both movements on the other side.

▶Benefits: Develops flexibility and strength in the hips and legs; improves balance.

Knee Lifts

From the mountain pose with feet
hip-width apart, alternately lift first
one knee as high as possible, and
then the other, maintaining an
erect spine. Keep the arms and
hands relaxed at the sides. Move
at a moderately vigorous pace for
15–20 seconds.

▶Benefits: Strengthens the hip flexor
muscles in the pelvis; develops
flexibility in the hip and knee joints.

Overhead Stretch

From the mountain pose, inhale and
as you rise onto the balls of the feet
lift the arms forward and overhead.
Exhale as you lower the heels and
the arms. Then inhale and as you lift
the arms to the sides and overhead,
again rise onto the balls of the feet.
Exhale and lower the arms to the
sides as you lower the heels. Repeat
this sequence for 12 breaths.

▶Benefits: Improves circulation,
balance, coordination; develops
flexibility in the shoulders and
strength in the lower legs.

Mountain Pose with
Crossed Arms (Tadasana)

Stand with your feet parallel and
hip-width apart. Let your spine be
erect and your weight balanced over
the arches of the feet. Fold your arms
at your chest and close your eyes.
Rest for 30–45 seconds, allowing
your breath to become smooth.

▶Benefits: Establishes a neutral,
balanced alignment of the body
that provides an inner reference for
standing and other poses. Brings
awareness to posture in daily life.

Knee Lifts

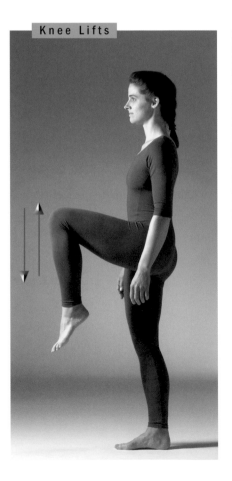

Overhead Stretch

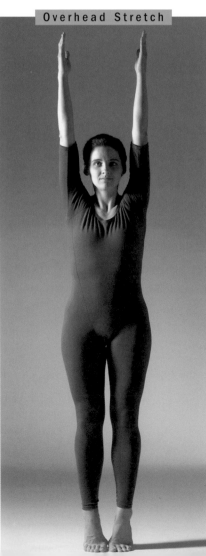

Mountain—Crossed Arms

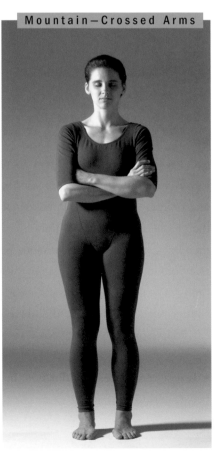

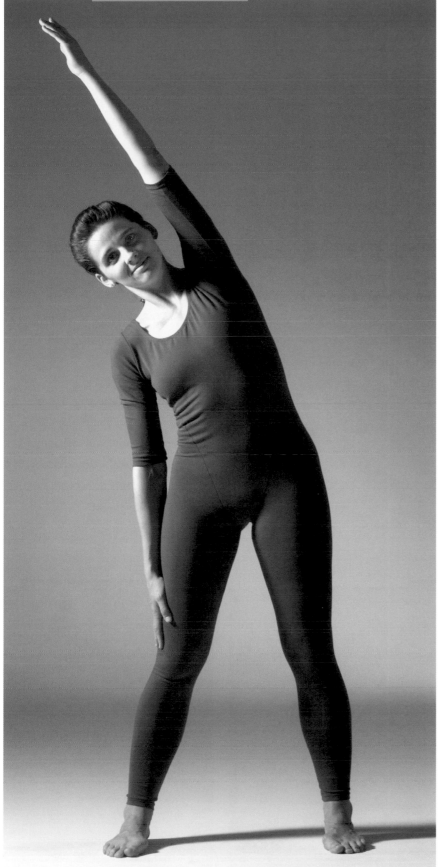

Standing Side Bend

Start with the feet 3 feet apart and parallel. Inhaling, raise the left arm to shoulder level, then turn the palm up and continue lifting the arm overhead. Reach up, lengthening the left side of the body, and begin bending to the right side. Do not tilt forward or backward; keep the left elbow straight. Let the right hand slide down the right leg, providing some support as you deepen the bend. Hold the stretch for 3 deep relaxed breaths. Then inhale as you lift back to center; exhale and release the arm. Alternate sides, repeating twice on each side.

▶Benefits: Provides a deep stretch of the muscles on the side of the torso.

Standing Forward Stretch

a) Stand erect and clasp your hands behind you. If possible bring the palms of the hands together and straighten the elbows, lengthening the arms toward the floor. Draw the shoulders back and press the shoulder blades toward each other; lift the arms slightly from the back and open the chest. Now, without rounding the back, bend forward from the hip joints until the hamstring muscles (in the back of the legs) are stretched.

b) Then bend the knees and return to the starting position. Keep the back flat as you bend forward, and as you come up. Keep the feet flat on the floor. Once the movement is smooth, repeat 10 or more times, deepening the hamstring stretch as you continue.

▶Benefits: Develops awareness of bending forward from the hip joints rather than the lower back; strengthens and protects the lower back while stretching the hamstring muscles.

Abdominal Squeeze
(Akunchana Prasarana)

Stand with the feet slightly wider than hip-width apart. Bend your knees and lean forward, placing the hands on the thighs. Settle the weight of the torso on the arms, relaxing the abdomen. Exhale and firmly contract the abdominal muscles, pressing the navel toward the spine. Then, as you inhale, relax and let the abdomen return to its normal position. Repeat 10 times.

▶Benefits: This important exercise for the abdomen tones, massages, and improves circulation to the abdominal organs, and strengthens the abdominal wall. Coordinates diaphragmatic breathing with abdominal movement.

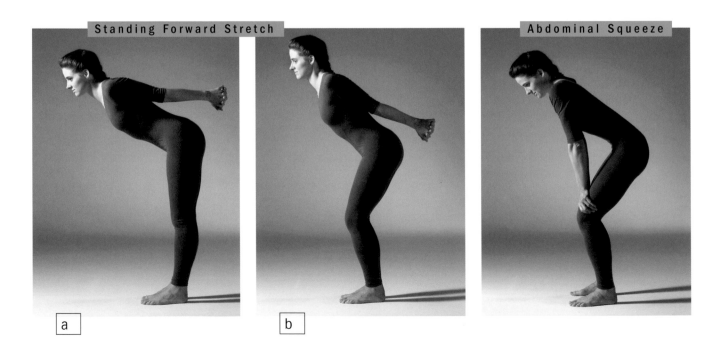

Standing Forward Stretch

a

b

Abdominal Squeeze

20

Forward Twisting Bend

Stand with the feet well apart. Raise the arms to the sides and bend
forward from the hip joints, keeping the lower back flat. Now twist to
the right and place the left hand on the right leg or on the floor in front
of the right foot (bend the knees if necessary). Raise the right arm above
you, turning the chest and head to look at that hand. Then, remaining in
the forward bend, reverse the twist, taking the right hand to the left side.
Slowly alternate sides 3–5 times. Breathe steadily throughout the movements,
exhaling as you deepen into the twist and inhaling as you release.

▶ Benefits: Stretches the hamstrings and inner thighs; develops flexibility
in the hips and spine; tones the abdomen; improves balance.

Forward Twisting Bend

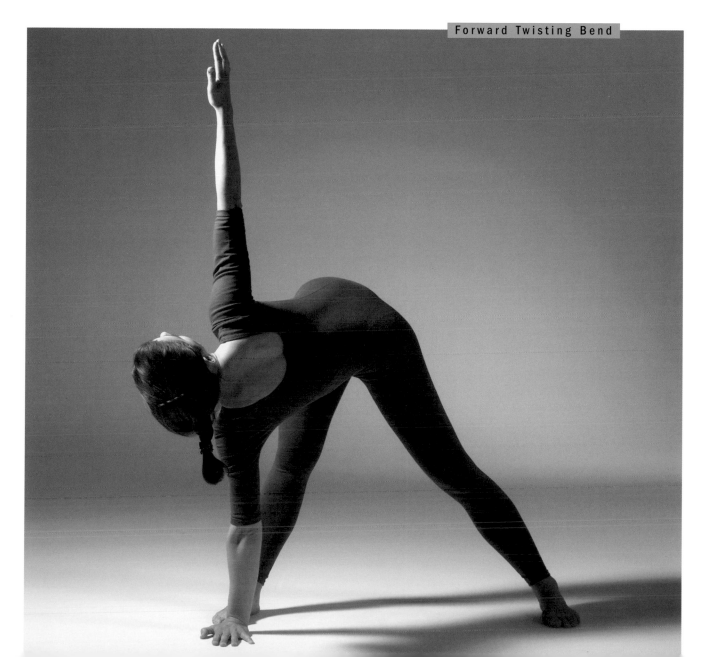

Cat Pose (Bidalasana)

a) Rest on your hands and knees, with the palms under the shoulders and the knees directly under the hips (the table pose). Exhaling, contract the abdominal muscles, tuck the pelvis, and round the spine, arching the back upwards.

b) Inhaling, release the abdominal muscles as you lift the sitting bones, spread the buttocks, lift the head, and arch the spine down. Keep the arms straight and the weight evenly distributed between the hands and knees. Repeat these two movements 5 times.

c) To further strengthen the back, with each inhalation extend and lift one leg straight behind you. Keep the two sides of the pelvis parallel to the floor.

d) Exhaling, curl the knee toward the forehead, arching the spine upwards. Repeat these two movements 5 times on each side.

Cat Pose

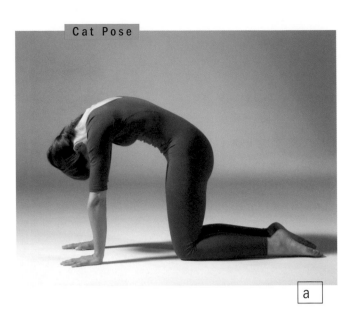

a

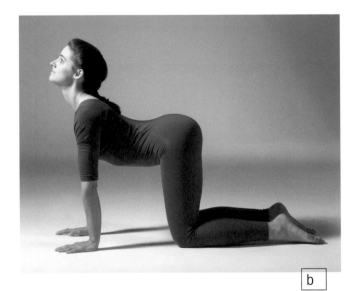

b

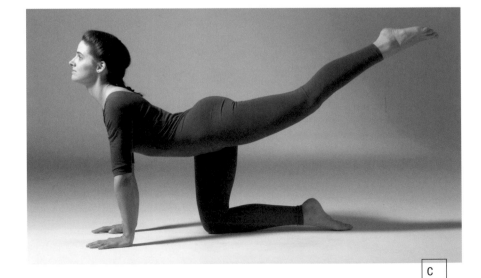

c

▶<u>Benefits</u>: Increases flexibility in
the spine; strengthens the abdomen;
tones the muscles of the back.

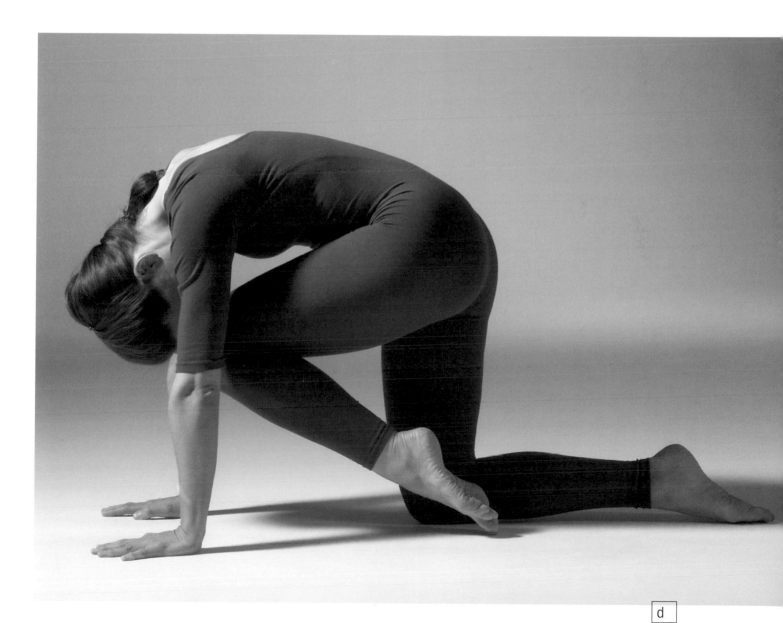

Extended Child's Pose (Balasana)

Sit on the heels with the toes touching. Place a cushion under your hips or ankles if you experience discomfort. Fold forward from the hips, stretching the arms overhead on the floor. While settling the weight back toward the hips, keep the arms straight as you stretch them forward. Walk the fingers away from the body to lengthen the arms. Hold and stretch for 5 breaths.

▶Benefits: Stretches the shoulders and back.

Cat Pose Balance

Return to your hands and knees. Extend and lift the left leg behind you with the toes extended, hips and leg parallel to the floor. Then raise the right arm parallel to the floor. Balance on the left hand and right knee while reaching out through the extended arm and leg. Release and repeat on the opposite side. Hold each side for 3–5 breaths.

▶Benefits: Strengthens the back; improves balance and coordination.

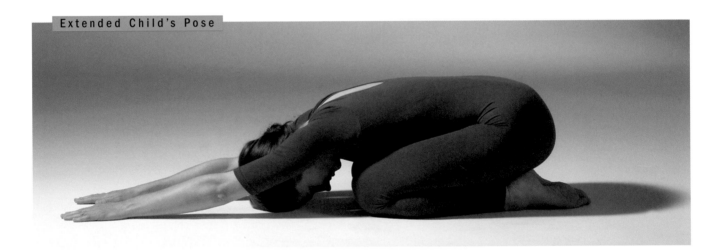

Extended Child's Pose

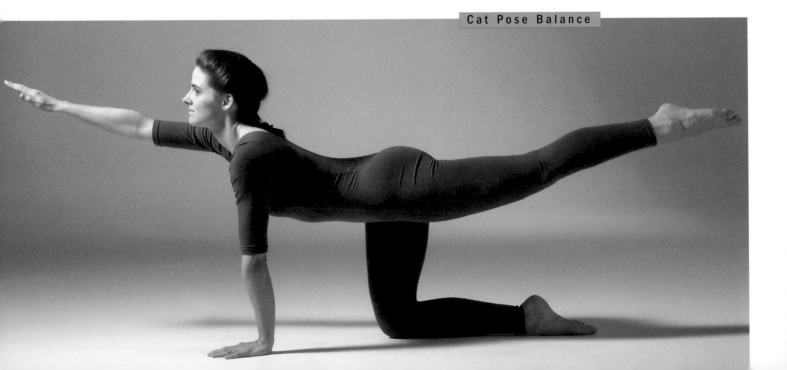

Cat Pose Balance

24

Cat Pose Twist

To twist while in the cat pose, shift the palm of the right hand to the left so that it is directly under your face. You may wish to spread the knees farther apart. Exhaling, twist to the left and raise the left arm. Open the chest, stretch up through the left arm, and turn the head to look at the hand. Inhale as you lower the arm. Repeat on the other side, holding the twist for 5 breaths on each side.

▶Benefits: Strengthens the back; improves balance and coordination; develops flexibility in the spine and shoulders.

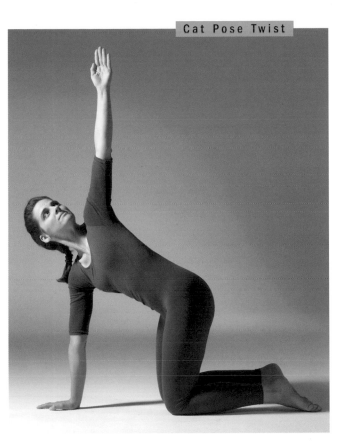
Cat Pose Twist

25

Lunge Pose (Banarasana)

Begin on your hands and knees, then step the left foot forward between the hands so that the toes are in line with the fingers. Extend the right leg straight behind, resting the knee and the top of the foot on the floor. Keep the left knee directly over the left ankle, with the shin perpendicular to the floor. Now lower the pelvis toward the floor, lengthening the two thighs in opposite directions, and pressing the front of the torso forward and gently up. Relax and lengthen the neck. Hold for 5 breaths. Then come back to the hands and knees and repeat on the other side.

▶Benefits: An important stretch for proper alignment of the pelvis. Stretches the hip flexor muscles deep in the pelvis, as well as the front of the thighs.

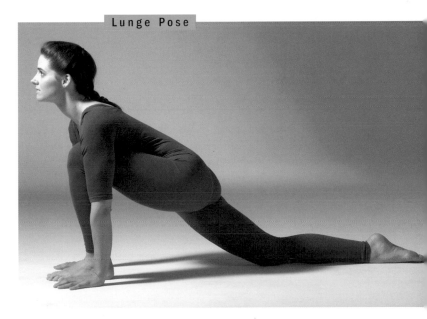
Lunge Pose

Cobra Pose (Bhujangasana)

a) Lie face down on the floor with the legs together. Place the palms flat on the floor just beyond the head, touching thumb to thumb and index finger to index finger. The elbows are comfortably bent. Firm the buttocks, hips, and legs.

b) Slide the nose forward, then begin to lift the head and chest. Press the forearms into the floor and draw the upper torso forward and up. Press down through the arms, lengthening and lifting the rib cage away from the pelvis and pressing the chest forward. Concentrate on lengthening the entire spine without stressing the lower back. Open the throat by drawing the shoulders down away from the ears to lengthen the back of the neck. Soften the eyes, face, and jaw. Experience the breath in the back of the waist and the sides of the rib cage as you hold the pose for 5 breaths.

Then exhale and lengthen down, extending and lowering the chest and chin to the floor first, then the nose, and finally tucking the head and bringing the forehead to the floor. Turn the head to one side, relax the arms alongside the body, and take a couple of resting breaths before continuing. You can repeat the pose, turning the head to the opposite side when you come out.

▶ Benefits: This important basic asana opens the chest, strengthens the upper back, increases flexibility and circulation in the upper spine, and tones the buttocks and lower back. Like other backward bends, the cobra pose dispels sluggishness, awakens vital energy, and freshens the mind. It also enhances breathing by releasing the tension in the chest and abdomen that keeps the diaphragm from moving freely and the lungs from expanding fully and evenly.

Cobra Pose

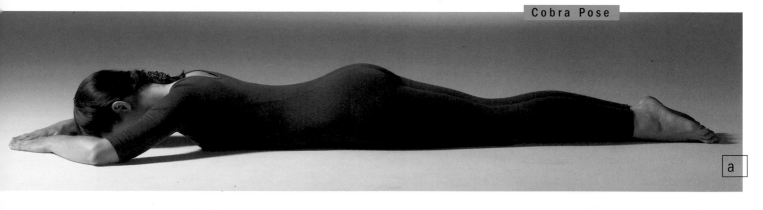

a

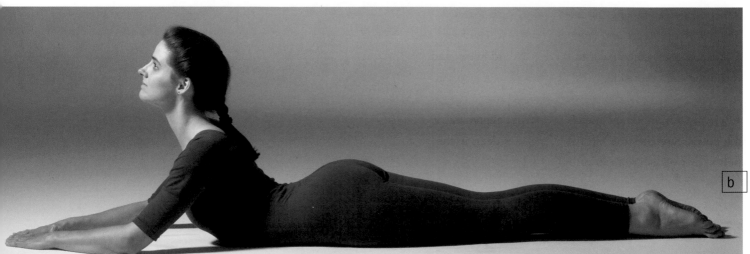

b

Boat Pose (Navasana)

a) Lie face down with the chin on the floor, legs together, and arms alongside the body, palms facing the hips. Lengthen the arms and draw the shoulder blades down the back. You will feel the abdomen expand against the floor as you inhale and contract as you exhale. Bring the legs firmly together and tighten the buttocks. Now, inhaling, press the lower abdomen into the floor as you lift both the legs and upper body. Keep the legs straight and the arms along the sides.

Lengthen the whole body, expand the chest, and allow the shoulders to move down and away from the ears. Hold the pose for 5 breaths and let the power of the inhalation and exhalation support you, riding the waves of the breath. Finally, exhale and release to the floor with the head turned to one side. Enjoy a few resting breaths, aware of the weight of the whole body on the floor.

b) Repeat the instructions above with the arms straight out to the sides at shoulder height, palms facing down. Be careful to keep the shoulders pulled down away from the ears, and to raise the chest as before.

c) The boat pose may also be done with arms overhead. Begin by coming into the pose with the arms extended to the sides at shoulder level. Inhaling, bring the arms parallel to one another alongside the ears with palms facing in. Lengthen the neck and let it be an extension of the spine. After 2–3 breaths release the posture by exhaling, opening the arms back out to the sides, and lowering the body to the floor. It is more difficult to bring the arms to the front and you may find that you won't lift quite as high as in the previous two versions.

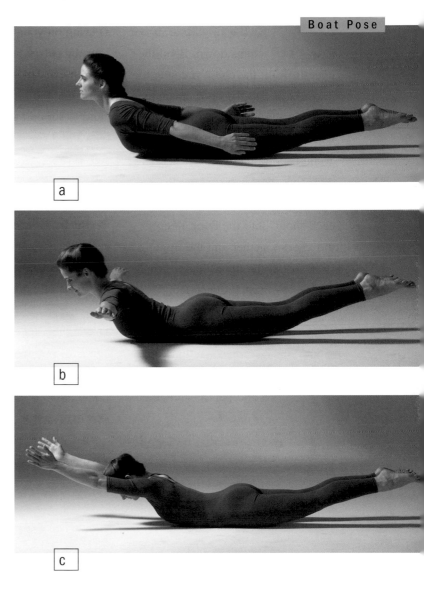

Boat Pose

a

b

c

▶Benefits: Strengthens the backside of the body; stimulates the abdomen and nervous system; improves circulation and overall body and breath awareness.

Rock Around the Clock

Curls

Lie on your back with your arms out to the sides, palms down. Bend the knees toward the chest, pressing the lower back into the floor. Imagine a clock on the backside of the pelvis with 12:00 at the tailbone and 6:00 at the back of the waist. Now rotate the pelvis clockwise around the rim of the clock, taking time to press each "hour" into the floor. Keep the knees together and the upper back flat on the floor. Begin with 5 rotations in each direction.

▶Benefits: Releases tension in the lower back; massages the back of the pelvis; improves circulation in the abdomen and pelvis; strengthens the abdominal muscles.

a) Lying on your back, bend the knees so that the feet are flat on the floor near the pelvis. Support the back of the head with the right hand. In one smooth exhalation curl the torso, bringing the head and knee toward each other. Use the strength of the abdomen to lift, grasping the knee with the left hand to support the movement. Avoid pulling on the head with the hand. Inhale and smoothly lower the foot and head to the floor. After 5 repetitions, switch to the other side and repeat 5 times.

b) Bend the knees and place both feet on the floor, placing the hands on the thighs. Exhale and curl the torso, bringing the head and knees toward each other. Again, use the strength of the abdomen to lift, grasping both knees with the hands to support the movement. Inhale and slowly lower to the starting position. Repeat 5 times.

c) Bend the knees and place both feet on the floor as before. Clasp the hands behind the head for support. Exhale and curl the torso, bringing the head and knees toward each other. Keep the elbows open to expand the chest. Avoid pulling on the neck and head with the hands. Inhale as you slowly release to the floor. Start with 5 repetitions.

▶Benefits: Strengthens the abdominal muscles.

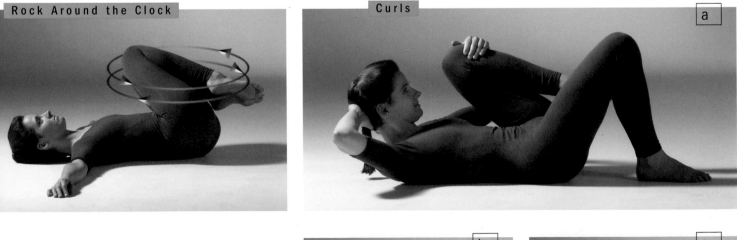

Rock Around the Clock

Curls

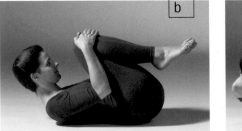

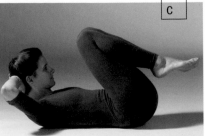

30

Inside Twist

Lying on your back with the knees bent, spread the feet and place them on the floor more than hip-width apart and near the pelvis. Stretch the arms out on the floor at shoulder level, palms down. Alternately bring one knee and then the other toward the floor near the opposite inner ankle. As one knee moves, the other remains upright. The shoulders and arms rest on the floor. Move continuously and rhythmically for 30 seconds.

▶ Benefits: Releases tension in the lower back.

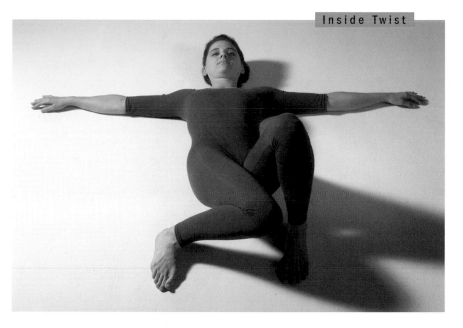

Inside Twist

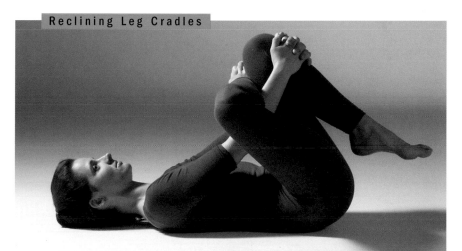

Reclining Leg Cradles

31

Reclining Leg Cradles

Lying on your back, bend the knees and bring the feet near the pelvis. Cross the right ankle at the left knee, pressing the right knee away. Lift the left thigh toward the abdomen. Slide the right arm between the thighs and interlace the hands at the back of the left thigh or around the shin. Continue to press the right knee away from the body as you draw the left thigh toward the abdomen. Rest the head on the floor (if it comes up off the floor, support it with a cushion), soften the face and jaw, and release resistance in the abdomen and deep muscles of the hip and buttock. The upper back and spine remain flat against the floor. Rock the left knee slowly from side to side or circle the knee to work more deeply into the stretch. Then breathe smoothly and relax, holding for 5–10 breaths. Repeat on the opposite side.

▶ Benefits: Increases hip flexibility; releases tension in the hip rotators; prepares the hips for sitting postures.

Couch Pose or Reclining Leg Stretch (Anantasana)

Lie on your right side with the right leg slightly bent for balance. Place your left foot on the floor in front of the pelvis, and prop your head with your right hand. With your left hand grasp your left big toe and straighten your leg upward, extending through the heel and drawing the toes toward the head.

    If you can't straighten the leg, grasp the ankle or shin, instead of the toes, and extend the leg as far as possible. Keep both sides of the torso long and the hips in line with the torso. Bend the knee and bring the foot back to the floor. Repeat several times, holding for 5 breaths the last time. Then repeat on the right side.

▶ <u>Benefits</u>: Stretches the hamstrings and improves balance.

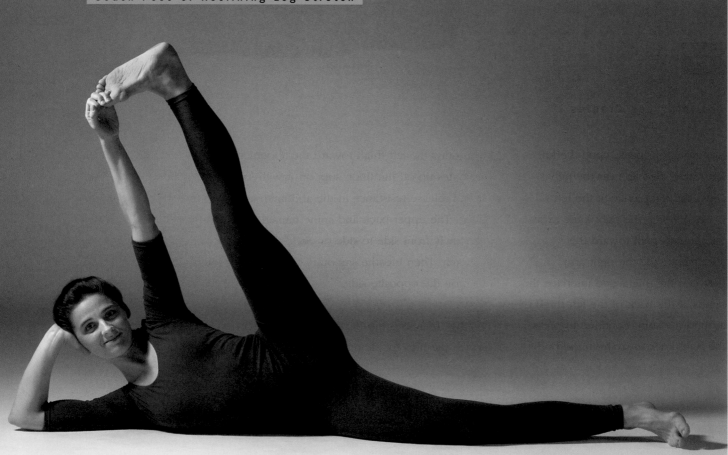

Couch Pose or Reclining Leg Stretch

33

Seated Forward Stretch (Churning)

a) Sit on the floor with the legs well apart, knees straight. Extend the heels and point the toes straight up.

b) Turn the torso to face the right leg and place the right hand on the floor behind and near the pelvis. Lift the lower back and bend from the hip joint toward the right leg, simultaneously sliding the left palm along the floor inside the right leg. Keep the lower back as long and flat as possible. Extend over the leg; then without pausing, lift slowly out of the stretch with a strong lower back. Change sides, bringing the left hand to the floor behind the pelvis and reaching the right arm and torso out to the left side. Repeat 5 times, alternating smoothly from side to side.

▶Benefits: Develops flexibility in the hips, mid- and lower back, and the back of the thighs; deepens the breath; prepares for seated forward bends.

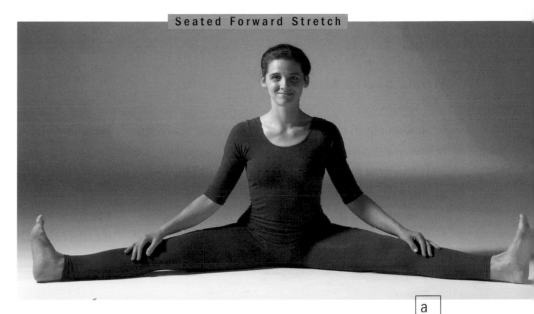

a

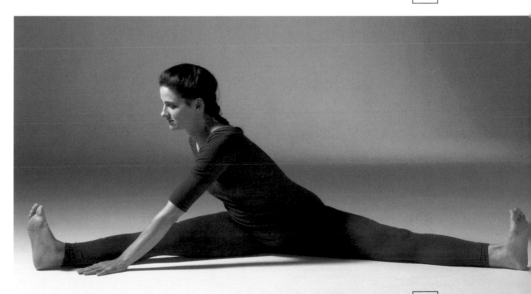

b

Simple Seated Twist

Sit in a simple cross-legged posture, each leg resting on or above the instep of the opposite foot. Keep the spine erect as you twist to the right, placing the fingertips of the right hand on the floor near the back of the pelvis and the left hand over the right knee. Breathe deeply, feeling the expansion and contraction of the abdomen and lower rib cage with each breath. Inhale and lengthen the spine, exhale and deepen the twist. Keep the shoulders down and level. Hold for 5–10 breaths. Then release and repeat on the opposite side.

▶ Benefits: Develops flexibility in the spine; strengthens the diaphragm; massages the abdomen; stretches the muscles of the shoulders and upper chest.

Simple Seated Twist

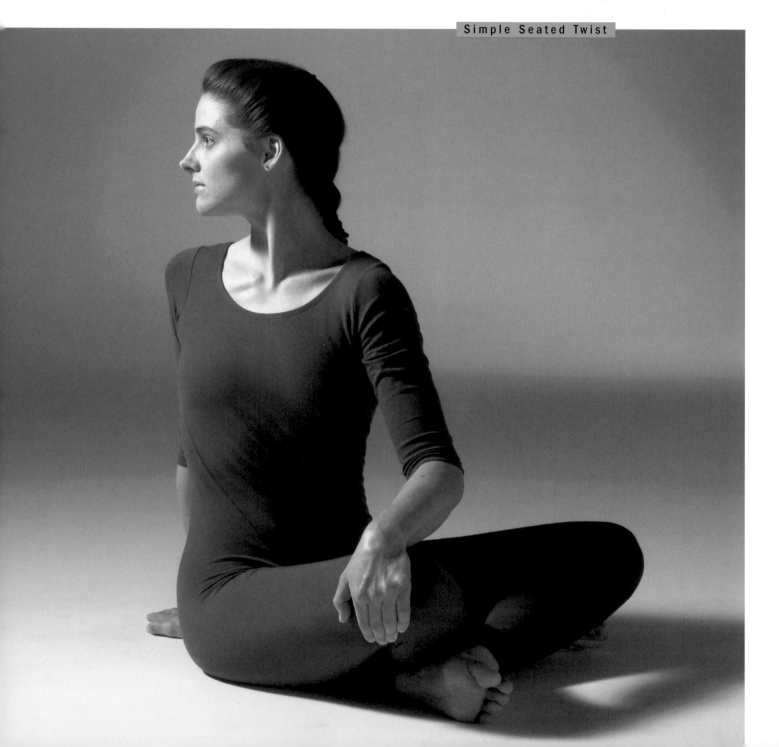

35

Rocking Chair

a) Sit on a carpeted surface or mat, knees raised and feet flat. Make sure there is space behind as well as in front of you. Clasp each thigh just behind the knee and round the entire spine (including the lower back) like a rocker on a rocking chair.

b) Keeping the spine rounded, gently roll backward toward the shoulders as you raise and straighten the legs. Then roll forward to the starting position, adding momentum by bending the knees. Be sure to keep the lower back rounded as you come forward, to make it easier to return to the upright position. Begin with 8–10 repetitions.

▶Benefits: Massages the back and spinal column; improves coordination and balance; prepares the body for inverted postures.

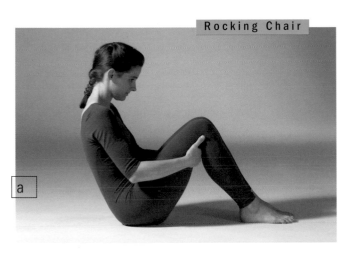

Rocking Chair

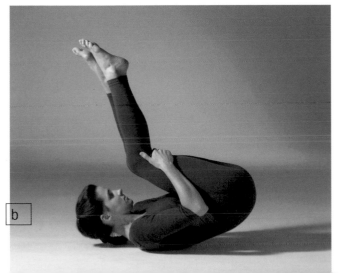

36

Folded Inversion

Roll backward from the upright rocking chair, keeping the knees bent. When you reach the shoulders, slide your hands from the thighs onto the lower back, placing the elbows on the floor. The hands support the pelvis and back. Bend the knees and rest the thighs above the abdomen. To deepen the stretch, shift the knees, placing them lightly on the forehead while adjusting the elbows for better support. Hold for 5 or more breaths.

Caution: Avoid this and all other inverted poses if you are menstruating or pregnant, if you have high blood pressure, glaucoma, a detached retina, or a neck injury, or if you have been advised against inverted poses for other reasons.

▶Benefits: Stretches muscles of the upper back and spine; increases circulation to the neck and head; relieves fatigue; improves concentration.

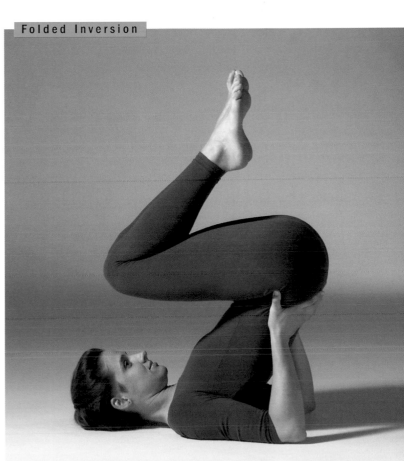

Folded Inversion

Reclining Twist Variation

Lie on your back, arms extended out to the side at shoulder level, palms down. Keeping the right leg straight on the floor, raise the left knee and place the left foot on the right knee. Twist the pelvis to the right. After turning halfway, lift the right hip and slide it further underneath to realign the torso and permit a deeper twist. Use the right hand on the left knee for additional leverage. Turn the head to the left, lengthen the left arm, and press the left shoulder toward the floor to deepen the twist. Breathe deeply in the stretch. Hold for 5–10 breaths. Repeat on the opposite side.

▶Benefits: Increases flexibility in the entire spine; massages and tones the abdomen; strengthens the diaphragm. This and the following two stretches relieve back discomfort.

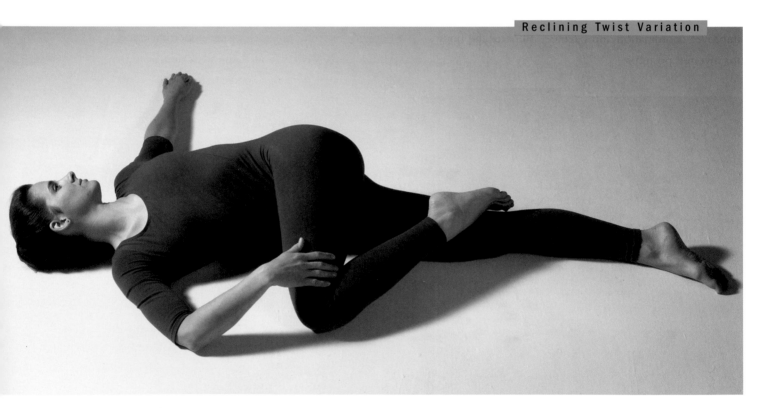

Reclining Twist Variation

Knees-to-Chest Pose (Pavanamuktasana)

a) Lie on your back, legs extended. Bend the right knee and clasp it with your hands, gently drawing the thigh toward the abdomen. Keep the pelvis and left leg on the floor. Hold the right knee securely but without straining, breathing smoothly and deeply. Rest the lower back firmly against the floor. Hold for 5–10 breaths, then repeat on the left side.

b) Next raise both knees, and clasping the hands around the legs, draw the thighs toward the abdomen. Again, gently press the lower back into the floor, relaxing the muscles there. Hold the pose, breathing evenly for 5–10 breaths.

▶Benefits: Releases lower back tension; massages the abdomen; flexes knee and hip joints.

Knees-to-Chest Pose

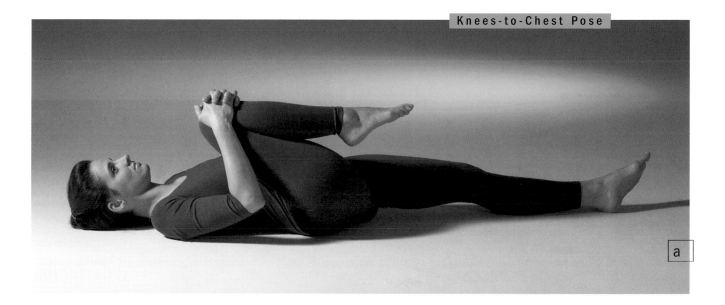

a

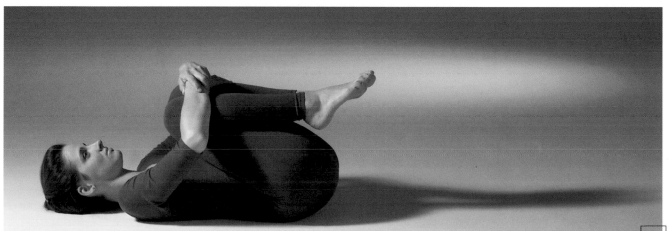

b

Pelvic Tilt

Lie on the back with the knees bent and the feet on the floor hip-width
apart. Rest the arms alongside the torso, palms down. Exhale and press the
lower back into the floor by contracting the abdominal muscles. Then slowly
lift the sacrum. Inhaling, release the abdominal contraction and lower the
pelvis back to the floor. Repeat 5 times.

Next, arch the spinal column higher. Contract the abdomen, press the
lower back into the floor, and curl the pelvis as before, but now continue
lifting, rolling up the spine one vertebra at a time. Start with the lower spine
and finally lift the chest, pressing the breastbone toward the chin. Return to
the floor by releasing slowly, one vertebra at a time, lengthening the lower
back and relaxing the buttocks. Throughout the movement keep the feet
pointed straight forward and pressed firmly and evenly into the floor. Repeat
5 times, or more, to release tension.

▶Benefits: Increases flexibility of the spine and pelvis; releases lower back
tension; develops more subtle control of the muscles of the lower back,
abdomen, thighs, and pelvis.

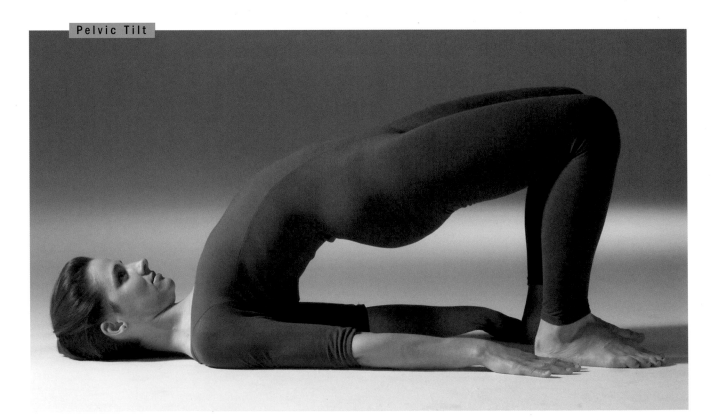

Pelvic Tilt

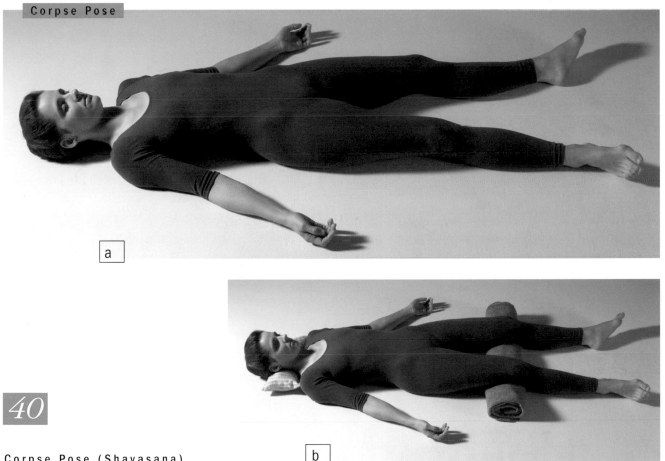

a

b

40

Corpse Pose (Shavasana)

a) Lie on your back on a firm, flat surface with a thin cushion to support the neck and head. Closing your eyes, lift and lengthen the back of the neck until the neck feels comfortable. Relax and lengthen the spine without bending to either side. Rest the legs about 12–14 inches apart. Rest the arms 6–8 inches from the sides, palms turned upward (they may, however, roll inward). Bring the shoulder blades slightly together, and draw them down toward the waist, opening the chest.

b) If there is discomfort in the lower back, support the back of the knees with a folded blanket or cushions. Cover the body with a light blanket for longer relaxations, or if you're chilly. Lie resting and observing the flow of your breath for 5–10 minutes. (You may wish to use one of the relaxation methods found in chapter 8.)

To come out of the relaxation, gently move your fingers and toes—then stretch the arms overhead on the floor as you stretch down through the legs. When you are ready bend the knees, roll over to the left side, and finally sit up. Sit quietly for a moment before continuing with the day.

▸Benefits: Integrates and consolidates the benefits of the other postures. Quiets the mind; restores energy; balances the nervous system. Eases strain on the heart by placing the entire body at the same level. Permits deep, relaxed breathing.

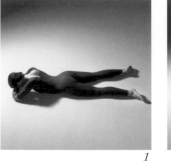

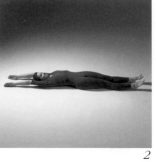

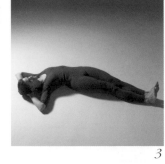

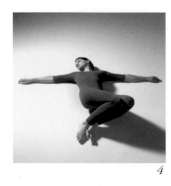

1 *2* *3* *4*

48

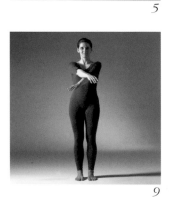

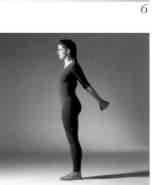

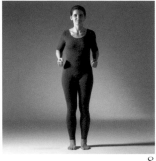

5 *6* *7* *8*

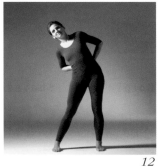

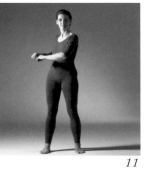

9 *10* *11* *12*

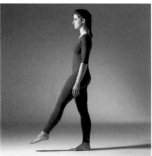

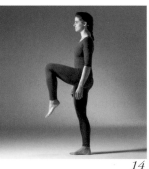

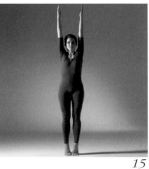

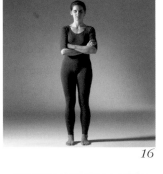

13 *14* *15* *16*

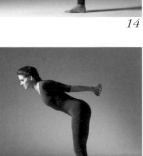

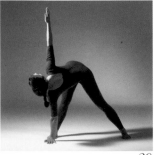

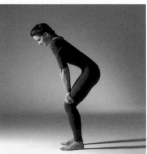

17 *18* *19* *20*

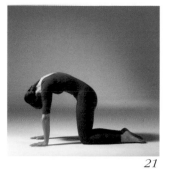
21

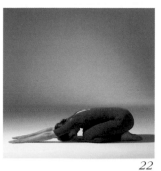
22

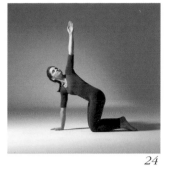
23

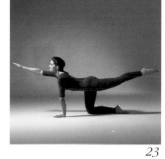
24

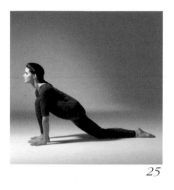
25

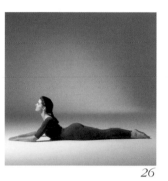
26

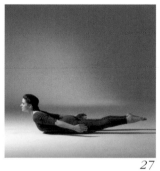
27

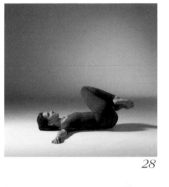
28

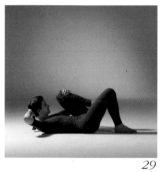
29

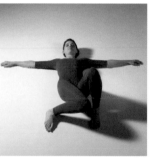
30

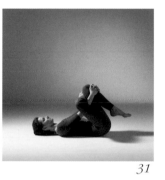
31

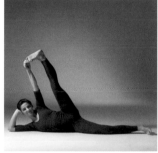
32

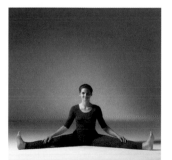
33

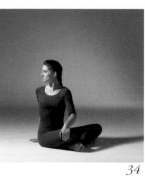
34

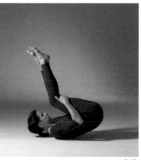
35

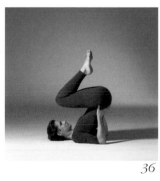
36

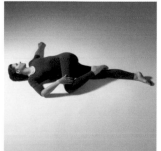
37

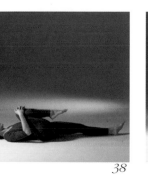
38

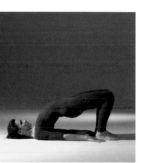
39

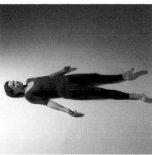
40

CHAPTER FOUR

TRAINING THE BREATH

When you observe that your breath is serene,
deep, and without any unnecessary pause,
you will experience a sense of great comfort and joy.
—— *Swami Rama*

AN ancient story, told in the *Chandogya Upanishad*, begins with a heated dispute among the eyes, ears, mind, and vital breath, over which is the most indispensable for human life. To resolve the issue each function agrees to vacate the body for one year, leaving the others to manage without it. After they have all returned, the function with the greatest importance will be determined.

One by one the eyes, the ears, and the mind depart— and through blindness, loss of hearing, and a nearly coma-like existence, life manages to continue. Then the vital breath begins to leave, and suddenly the remaining functions find themselves uprooted as if a strong horse, anchored to the ground, were pulling up the stakes that held it. Awestruck, the other senses beseech the breath to return, humbly accepting its preeminent role in sustaining life.

Despite its profound importance, for the most part breathing is a background to other activities; its ceaseless flow remains on the periphery of our awareness. A noxious smell, something entering the windpipe by mistake, or a thick cloud of dust forces us to pay momentary attention to it, but when problems are resolved the breath recedes into the background once again. We are not aware that it is embedded in our every thought and movement.

It is convenient that we don't have to constantly monitor the breath, but this can have unintended consequences. Frequently—and often from an early age—poor breathing habits, misalignments in body posture, and muscle imbalances undermine the breath's effectiveness. Low energy levels, shortness of breath, anxiety, stress, and poor concentration are just some of the resulting symptoms.

These conditions can be reversed, and you will learn the beginning steps for doing so in the following pages, which explain the mechanics of the breath and include illustrations of the basic muscles of respiration. They describe five techniques for improving your style of breathing so that with proper training your breath can be strong, healthy, and relaxed—and you will enjoy a higher level of well-being.

Natural Control of Breathing

The normal tempo of the breath is slow. On average, the heart beats 70 times in a minute, while we breathe just 16 times. Yet these 16 breaths mean that the lungs expand and contract over 20,000 times per day, consuming about 35 pounds of air—6 times the weight of our daily intake of food and liquids.

The rate of breathing varies throughout the day. After vigorous exercise it may increase to well over 30 breaths per minute, and during meditation it may slow to as little as 5 or fewer. Throughout this fluctuation its rhythmic pulsing maintains the integrity of body and mind.

The autonomic nervous system is responsible for regulating breathing as well as other essential functions such as heartbeat and body temperature. These are all automatically controlled by this system, and normally such internal processes operate unconsciously. Breathing, however, is unique in that it is carried out with skeletal muscles that can be brought to conscious awareness. For example, if you wish to breathe out quickly, inhale more deeply, or briefly hold your breath— you can at will.

And because breathing is the only autonomic function that can be accessed in this way, it plays an enormously important role in the self-regulation techniques of yoga, for it is through the apparently fragile (but ultimately strong) thread of breath that entrance is gained to the inner dimensions of the psyche where balance, peace, and stability can prevail in the face of tension and stress.

Breathing and the Autonomic Nervous System

Stress creates an imbalanced and overloaded nervous system. During stressful times our thoughts reflect the fear and uncertainty we encounter in daily life, and in one way or another they conclude, "I can't handle this." The mind and nervous system react with heightened arousal, followed by fatigue, and ultimately illness as the stress wears on. Then, if attempts to resolve the tension are not successful, the smooth integration of the nervous system begins to break down. Body cues such as hunger are not recognized and are replaced with sporadic or nervous eating; movement is clumsy; there are changes in body temperature; our attention vacillates. These and many other changes are traced to "my nerves."

The breath is a barometer for the nervous system; as it becomes imbalanced, breathing changes as well, becoming shallow, tense, jerky, and marked by notable sighs and pauses. This in turn is registered by the mind, and an internal feedback loop is established. Changes in breathing create internal distress, which sustains poor breathing, which sustains distress…. Thus stress takes on a life of its own; it exists apart from the stressor that originally triggered the reaction.

Relaxed diaphragmatic breathing—yogic breathing— is a powerful aid to restoring nervous system coordination and harmony. Inner tensions soften as the breath returns to its natural rhythm, and the loss of control that often accompanies stress is diminished. Most important, each relaxed breath calms the mind and enables us to recover strength and the will to go forward.

The Breath in Daily Life

The condition of the nervous system, the state of emotional life, and the quality of breathing are closely related. Events that take place in the outer environment as well as in the mind are all registered in the breath. For example, if a car directly ahead of yours were to suddenly stop, you might very well gasp sharply as you slam on the brakes; and during an intense workweek even the thought of a weekend off brings a sigh of relief. We breathe in sharply when we are startled, sigh when we are sad (or in love), and laugh by distinctively starting and stopping the exhalation. When an emotion is painful we may shut down our feelings by restricting the breath; when an emotion is pleasant we breathe slow and easy. All these changes in the pattern of breathing momentarily amplify our reactions.

When agitated breathing is prolonged it creates an unsettled and defensive outlook on life. Relaxed breathing, on the other hand, calms the nervous system. When the breath is habitually deep and smooth, reactions to life events do not create marked disturbances in our emotional life. This is why relaxed breathing has been used to good effect in the treatment of cardiovascular disease, panic/anxiety, migraine headaches, hypertension, and asthma. And most important, from the point of view of mental health the relationship between breathing and

emotion is a two-way street: relaxed breathing can calm even highly agitated emotions during periods of distress; it helps maintain a cheerful contentment when life is going well.

Breathing in Yoga Practice

Yogis have learned to work with the breath in many ways. Strenuous postures, or those that require holding the body in awkward positions, clearly reveal the calming effect of relaxed breathing. When we encounter such challenging postures we either adapt to them if the breathing is relaxed or struggle against them by altering the breath. In other words, relaxed breathing has an influence throughout the entire period of asana practice and plays an enormous role in its effectiveness.

In yoga breathing exercises, or pranayama practices, the breath is used to cleanse, calm, and strengthen the nervous system, and thus increase vitality. What is more, adepts in yoga have demonstrated abilities that go far beyond the normal capacity for controlling the breath, yet they do not claim to be superhuman. They simply state that the full potential of breath control is much vaster than is normally experienced and cannot be understood without patient practice.

The breath is also a key focal point in relaxation exercises as well as meditation. However, because relaxation is usually practiced lying down (either on the back or on the stomach), while meditation is practiced in a sitting position, the breathing pattern differs in each posture. So we must thoroughly understand the principles of relaxed breathing in order to master these essential practices.

Breathing can also strengthen the mind's powers of concentration. At first relaxation and meditation techniques use the breath as a tool for centering attention. Later, when breathing has become effortless, relaxed, and smooth, the mind is freed from all distractions and can turn inward toward deeper levels of awareness.

Breath training is a systematic process. The skills taught in this chapter lead to a strong, healthy breath and constitute a solid foundation for yoga. The following list summarizes them. You will want to return to it from time to time to review your progress.

Step One: Learn to practice sustained breath awareness, observing the breath as it flows in and out.

Step Two: Form the habit of breathing through the nose.

Step Three: Learn to recognize the sensations associated with diaphragmatic breathing, and breathe diaphragmatically in the corpse pose, the crocodile pose, and a sitting pose.

Step Four: Strengthen the diaphragm.

Step Five: Practice five qualities of good breathing, letting the breath be (1) deep, (2) smooth, (3) even, (4) without sound, and (5) without pause.

STEP ONE: BREATH AWARENESS

The first step in breath training is to cultivate a sustained awareness of the breath as it flows in and out. Yoga stretches and postures can help you accomplish this, as the following series of simple movements will make clear.

Stand erect with your arms alongside your body, your feet hip-width apart and parallel to one another. As you inhale, lift the arms out to the sides. Exhaling, let the arms come down. Do this a number of times to feel the coordination of breath and movement.

Next, inhale and continue the movement until the arms are parallel to one another over your head. Exhaling, lower the arms back to the sides. Again, repeat the movement a number of times to make the coordination of breath and movement natural.

Finally, lift the arms over your head and hold them there, clasping the palms together. Although you are holding the stretch, do not hold your breath; continue to breathe out and in without pause, maintaining your awareness of the breath. If you relax your abdomen you will feel a dramatic expansion and contraction there and at the sides of the rib cage. These movements are the result of deep breathing. When you are ready, exhale and lower the arms.

Coordinating your breathing with the movement of your body heightens breath awareness and produces a more relaxed stretch. It will improve your understanding of the muscles of breathing, deepen the breath, identify and relax unconscious muscle resistance, and calm your mind.

Cleansing and Nourishing

As you observe your breathing, you will notice that the inhalation and exhalation serve different purposes. When the breath flows in, it carries energy along with it, revitalizing the body and mind. When the breath flows out, it gathers the wastes that the blood has brought to the lungs, and bears them away. The inhalation is invigorating; the exhalation usually requires little effort and is relaxing.

A tranquil, steady awareness of this process plays an important part in virtually every aspect of yoga practice, so get into the habit of doing the following exercise each morning and evening. It will soon become a foundation for other breathing exercises as well as for relaxation and meditation. It will also provide an experience you can return to at times of stress and tension.

EXERCISE: Relaxed Breath Awareness

You might try recording this and the other four exercises that follow. Read them aloud into a recording device at a slow pace; then play them back as you practice.

▶ Lie in the corpse pose on a firm, flat surface. Close your eyes and let your body rest. Take a few minutes to adjust to the stillness of your posture. The floor will support you, and you can release into it.

▶ When you are ready, bring your awareness to the flow of your breathing. Feel the breath flowing out and then flowing in. As the breath flows out, it cleanses, carrying away wastes and fatigue. As the breath flows in, it draws in fresh energy and a sense of well-being.

▶ Soften the abdomen, releasing tension there and allowing it to rise and fall with each breath. Relax the muscles of the rib cage. Let the breath flow without pausing after the exhalation or after the inhalation. Again and again observe the flow of the two streams of breath. Recognize the difference in the sensations associated with the exhalation and inhalation. Become familiar with your breathing without trying to judge whether you are breathing "correctly." Just feel the two streams of breath.

▶ Remain resting and aware of the breath for 5 minutes. You may find that your mind relaxes and your nervous system becomes more calm, and if this happens just let it happen, without any attachment to it. Simply continue watching the flow of the breath. Then, when you are rested, slowly cup your eyes with your palms, open your eyes to your hands, stretch your body, roll to your side, and come back to a sitting position.

You will find that the process of watching the breath affects the mind—it gradually relieves the frenetic pace of thinking, and a calm focus develops. Each exhalation feels relaxing, and each inhalation feels nourishing. With practice it will soon be possible to bring your awareness to your breathing at other times of the day, when you are not doing the formal exercise in the corpse pose. For example, you can practice breath awareness while you are out for a walk or working out on exercise equipment. It is a very versatile tool for centering and calming emotional tensions.

In Case of Anxiety

This breathing exercise, as well as the others in this chapter, relaxes the flow of breathing and is usually restful. Rarely, however, some students report feeling nervous about watching the breath. If this is the case for you, don't give up. You might try the exercise sitting in a comfortable chair— or lying down with the eyes open for a time. A few attempts is usually all it takes to get over the jitteriness and turn the experience into a pleasant one.

STEP TWO: BREATHING THROUGH THE NOSE

In Sanskrit the nasal area is called *sapta-patha,* meaning "seven paths," because it is the confluence of seven openings: the two nostrils, the two tear ducts, the two Eustachian tubes, and the pharynx (the upper throat). In addition, the sinuses are connected to the nose through small orifices. Filtered, warmed, cleaned, moistened, and tested for noxious smells, air passing inward through the nose is strikingly transformed by its brief sojourn in this area.

The nose, sinuses, and nasal pharynx are lined with highly sensitive tissue containing two special cell types: goblet and ciliated cells. Goblet cells secrete mucus. Ciliated cells contain tiny hair-like filaments that beat rhythmically to move the mucus from the nose into the throat, where it can be swallowed (or spit out).

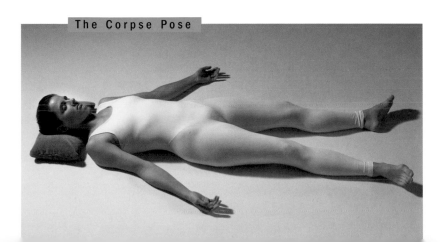

The Corpse Pose

From the yogic point of view mucus can be either a healthy secretion or an unpleasant excretion. A healthy blanket of mucus traps airborne particles carried into the nose—including microbes that can cause disease. A healthy mucus lining also lubricates the nose and moistens the air, which otherwise can be extremely drying (as you can appreciate when it becomes necessary to breathe through the mouth).

Three shelf-like structures of bone (turbinates) and tissue (conchae) extend into the space within the nose. The air whirls by them, increasing its contact with the mucus lining and improving the senses of smell and

taste. In addition, the conchae alternately swell and shrink in size, which changes the balance of air flowing through the two nostrils.

Breathing through the mouth bypasses all of these important warming, moistening, and filtering functions, and should therefore be done only at peak times of effort when the body's need for oxygen requires a rapid exchange of air. Otherwise, breathing in and out through the nose is by far the best choice.

Some students have learned to breathe in through the nose and out through pursed lips while they are exercising. This technique activates the abdominal muscles and brings awareness to them, but it is not generally used in yoga or for normal, everyday breathing. Exhaling through the nose results in a prolonged exhalation that balances the length of the inhalation and maintains open bronchial passageways for the duration of the breath.

Unfortunately, congestion in the nose can prevent the air from flowing easily, and when that is the case a simple method of cleansing the nose, the neti wash (described in chapter 7), can provide relief. If the nose is chronically congested, however, it may be helpful to consult with a healthcare provider because congestion of this kind can result from a variety of causes.

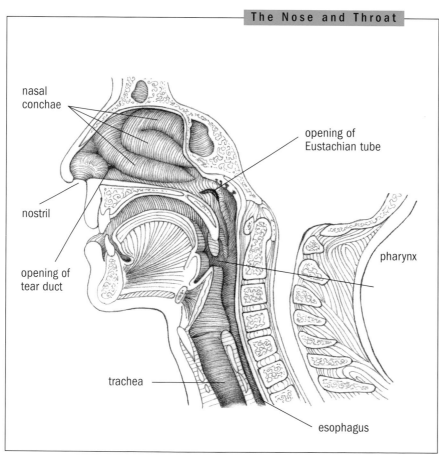

The Nose and Throat

nasal conchae

opening of Eustachian tube

nostril

opening of tear duct

pharynx

trachea

esophagus

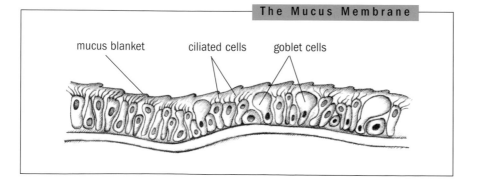

The Mucus Membrane

mucus blanket · ciliated cells · goblet cells

To gain firsthand knowledge of the difference between breathing through the mouth and the nose, you may want to try a very simple experiment. Take 5–10 breaths each to compare the feeling of breathing through the nose with the feeling of breathing through an open mouth. Observe the length, depth, and style of the breath, as well as its effect as it touches the membrane in the nose and mouth. Determine for yourself if breathing through the nose really does feel better.

STEP THREE: BREATHING WITH THE DIAPHRAGM

The lungs, unlike the heart, are not made of muscle fibers, and for this reason they cannot breathe by themselves. Embedded in the chest, they are connected to the air surrounding the body by a passageway through the nose and throat. And since they have no ability to force air through this tube, the lungs are like guests at a banquet being served to them by assistants. The assistants, in this case, are the various muscles of respiration. To put it awkwardly, we must "breathe the lungs." The choice of muscles we use to do this, and our ability to use these muscles skillfully, makes all the difference in the quality of our breathing.

The primary muscle of breathing is the diaphragm, and when it is functioning normally it accounts for about 75 percent of the volume of each inhalation. Unfortunately, bad breathing habits abound, and often the diaphragm's functioning gets restricted, or partially supplanted by other muscles.

There are a number of techniques for regaining the feeling of strong, diaphragmatic breathing. A brief review of the mechanisms of respiration is a good place to start, and after this review anatomical images can be translated into personal experience.

The Diaphragm

The diaphragm is a dome-shaped muscle lying below the lungs. Underneath the dome are the organs of the abdomen, and above it are the lungs and heart. The diaphragm thus divides the torso into two separate chambers. Blood vessels and the digestive tract pass through the diaphragm, but otherwise the organs above and below have no direct contact.

Like every skeletal muscle, the diaphragm contracts when it is stimulated by nerve impulses—and inhalation takes place. Then, as the nerve impulses diminish, the diaphragm relaxes, exhalation takes place, and air leaves the lungs. Exhalation is the result of a combination of forces, the most important of which is the natural elasticity of the lung tissue, which causes the lungs to contract when they are no longer stimulated to expand. As a result exhalation is usually a passive process, and when you sit down in a comfortable chair to relax, you will most likely exhale.

If necessary, muscle contractions in the abdomen and in the chest wall can increase the force of the exhalation. When you blow up a balloon or blow into your palms on a cold day, for example, you can feel additional

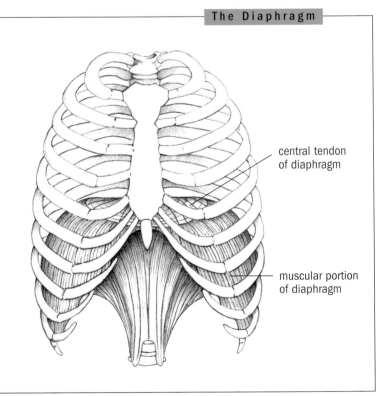

The Diaphragm

central tendon
of diaphragm

muscular portion
of diaphragm

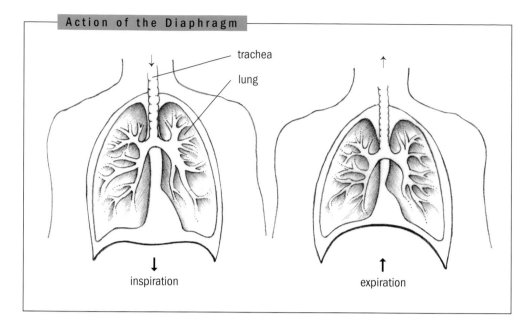

Action of the Diaphragm

trachea

lung

↓
inspiration

↑
expiration

pressure from the abdominal muscles during the exhalation. (A number of breathing exercises in yoga make use of this additional force, and one of these will be discussed in chapter 7.)

The Diaphragm in Action

The diaphragm is not made entirely of muscle tissue. The middle portion, lying just beneath the lungs, is called the central tendon and consists of relatively inflexible, leathery connective tissue. The muscular portions of the diaphragm slope down from the central tendon, and when these contract they pull the central tendon down. This, in turn, pulls the base of the lungs downward, and inhalation takes place.

The organs below the diaphragm are tightly packed into the abdomen, and when the diaphragm descends these organs are squeezed from above. Seeking more space, and with virtually no place to go, they press outward. Depending upon the position of your body, this can be observed in the abdomen, in the lower ribs, or even in the back. Three common yoga positions illustrate this: the corpse pose (lying on the back), the crocodile pose (lying on the stomach), and any of the erect, seated postures. Read through the following brief explanations, then go on to the practice sections to try each of them for yourself.

The Corpse Pose

In the corpse pose the rib cage is virtually motionless, and the abdominal organs are squeezed toward the front of the body with each inhalation. You will feel your navel region rise each time you inhale and fall as you exhale, and for this reason it is often called "abdominal breathing" or "belly breathing." This is the first style of breathing taught in yoga classes, because all breathing is improved significantly when tension in the abdomen is unblocked and accessory muscles of breathing in the chest are rested.

In the exercise on page 55 you practiced simple breath awareness in the corpse pose. Using this as a foundation, now you can further shape your breathing so that alterations in natural breathing patterns caused by physical and mental tensions can be relieved and replaced by a deep, diaphragmatic breath.

EXERCISE: Diaphragmatic Breathing in the Corpse Pose

▶ Return to the corpse pose, supporting the head and neck with a thin cushion. Breathe through the nose.

▶ Keeping the elbows on the floor, place one hand at the navel and the other on the chest. Bring your awareness to your breath, and feel the flow of the exhalations and inhalations.

▶ Soften the abdomen so that it is free to move. Rest the muscles of the rib cage. Soon you will observe the characteristic rise and fall of the abdomen, and the almost complete stillness of the rib cage. That is the sign of diaphragmatic breathing in this posture.

(Note that the diaphragm itself cannot be felt directly with the hand since the diaphragm lies deep within the torso.)

► As you continue, gently regulate the movement of breathing until it becomes relaxed and effortless. You are not puffing up the abdomen to make it rise: it simply rises as the result of your inhalation. Each breath feels about the same; the rise and fall of the abdomen is repeated again and again with little change in the breath.

► Pay attention to the process. If you find yourself opening your mouth, or if the movement tends to shift to the chest, to become shallow, or to stop, you will need to make a more conscious effort to breathe deeply and smoothly—to expand the abdomen with each breath.

► Next, place the arms on the floor alongside your torso, and continue to observe the breath. Now watch the transitions between the breaths. As you come to the end of the inhalation and the abdomen has expanded, simply relax, and let the exhalation begin. At the end of the exhalation, relax, and let inhalation begin. Relaxing allows each exhalation to flow naturally into the next inhalation. There is no pause in its flow, and the cycle of breathing is continuous.

► Lie resting, observing this deep, relaxed breath for about 10 minutes. You may find that with regular practice even the modest effort needed to keep the breath flowing deeply and without pause can be relaxed. Watch the flow of your own breathing like a comfortable, detached observer—one who remains self-aware and inwardly content—whose focus is the movement of the breath.

► Finally, when you are ready, bring your awareness back to your whole body, stretch in any way that feels comfortable to you, roll to your side, and return to a sitting posture.

The Crocodile Pose

Relaxed diaphragmatic breathing is not always as easy to achieve as the previous exercise suggests. If you are accustomed to using chest muscles for breathing, for example, or if it feels odd to expand the abdomen as you inhale, or if you become nervous watching your breath and consequently lose your inner focus, then you will want to practice breathing in the crocodile pose. In fact, every student will benefit from practice in this pose. It is the key posture for centering your attention and fostering diaphragmatic breathing.

There are several versions of the crocodile pose, each helpful, and each designed to accommodate students at different levels of flexibility. We will use the posture illustrated below: the arms are folded and the head rests on the forearms; the chest is elevated by the arms; the

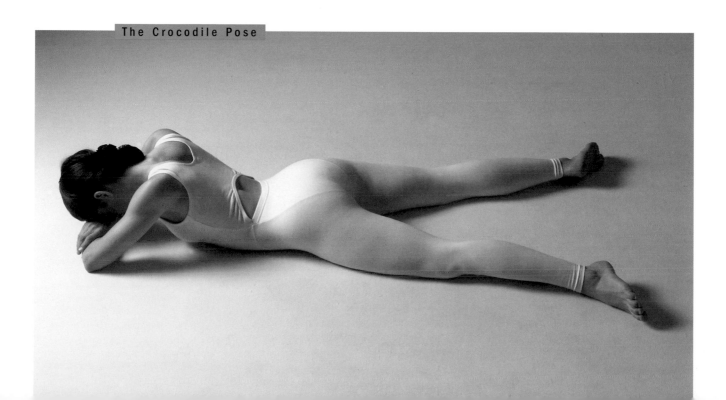

The Crocodile Pose

abdomen rests on the floor; and the legs are relaxed, either together or apart. If this is uncomfortable, you may modify the posture by placing a blanket or cushion beneath your upper chest and throat for support (drape your chin over the blanket so that you can breathe through the nose). You may also widen the elbows and partially open the forearms, allowing the hands to move toward one another (but do not lower the arms to your sides, as this will defeat the purpose of the pose).

The arms are raised above the level of the shoulders in the crocodile pose, which stretches and partially immobilizes the muscles in the chest. This requires the diaphragm to become more active. (Notice that with each breath the upper chest remains relatively still while the mid-torso expands and contracts.) What is more, when you are resting on your stomach and breathing diaphragmatically, the lower back and the sides of the rib cage expand, as does the abdomen. The lower back rises with the inhalation, and falls with the exhalation. The sides of the rib cage, and most notably the floating ribs, expand laterally with inhalation and return with exhalation. And since the muscles in both these areas are often chronically tense, stretching them during inhalation can feel refreshing. After experimenting a bit with your basic posture, continue with the following exercise.

EXERCISE: Diaphragmatic Breathing in the Crocodile Pose

► Lie on your stomach in the crocodile pose.

► Closing your eyes, let your body rest and become still. Gradually bring your awareness to your breathing. As you have done before, feel the movement of the breath as it ceaselessly flows out and in. The breath will find its own pace, and even if you believe the speed to be too fast or too slow, you don't need to control it. Simply observe your breath without judgment.

► As you continue to breathe, bring your attention to your lower back for several breaths. Feel the back rise as you inhale, and fall as you exhale. Next,

observe how the sides of the lower rib cage expand and contract with each breath. Finally, notice the pressure of the abdomen against the floor as you inhale, and the release of the abdomen as you exhale.

► After relaxing and observing the breath for some time you may want to deepen it further. Start by bringing your awareness to your navel region and see if perhaps you can soften that area even more than you already have. This calms the nervous system and reduces emotional tensions, and some find that this practice alone is helpful. It can be continued over a number of sessions or even weeks.

► You might also wish to try this experiment: at the end of the exhalation, breathe out a little more than usual by continuing to press the abdomen toward the spine. Then, as you slowly inhale, soften the muscles of the lower back and abdomen, and let the back rise and expand. You may feel as if the lower back is being stretched by the deep inhalation. Repeat the extra exhalation and the expanded inhalation for 5–10 breaths until you become accustomed to the feeling of the deep inhalation. Then return to your normal exhalation—but continue to let the lower back expand as you inhale. Your breath will feel slower and deeper.

► Remain resting in the crocodile pose for about 5 minutes. When you are refreshed, come out of the posture slowly, creating a smooth transition back to normal breathing.

Sitting and Standing Postures

When the body is erect, breathing movements shift noticeably to the sides of the lower ribs. So let's take a closer look at the mechanics of the rib cage in order to understand what is happening.

Even though the rib cage can be moved by various sets of muscles, its bony structure gives it a certain rigidity. As we have seen, when we are lying on our back in the corpse pose the rib cage is quiet and the abdomen rises and falls with minimal involvement of the rib cage. But when we are in an upright posture

Pump-Handle Motion of the Sternum

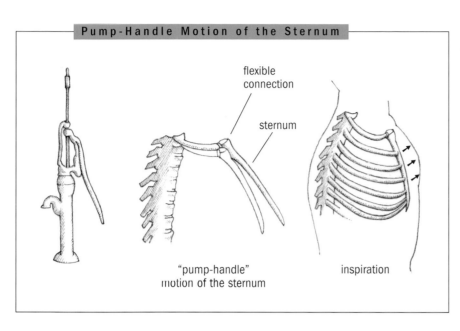

flexible connection

sternum

"pump-handle" motion of the sternum

inspiration

Bucket-Handle Motion of the Ribs

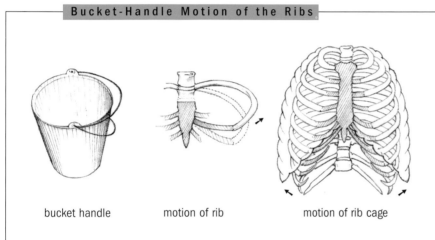

bucket handle   motion of rib   motion of rib cage

they are intended to provide sudden bursts of energy, but they are not meant for normal, everyday use. When either of these styles of breathing becomes habitual, emotional tension is increased, and this leads to feelings of anxiety as well as unnecessary stress.

An even more unfortunate breathing style can develop when the basic principles of breathing are not understood. You may have been told by a well-meaning friend that when you inhale you should expand your chest and pull your abdomen in. This, of course, will create tension in the lower abdomen and focus all your breathing efforts in your chest. It will lead to paradoxical breathing (in which the abdomen is compressed instead of expanded during inhalation), and this further exaggerates feelings of tension and anxiety.

The normal movement of the rib cage is far less extreme. During routine, moderate breathing in an

(sitting or standing) the ribs become more active, and two primary movements of the rib cage are possible.

First, during a very deep breath the sternum can be pulled forward and raised by intercostal muscles in the chest and by accessory muscles in the neck and shoulders—something like the movement of an old-fashioned pump handle. Joints near the top of the sternum make this possible. To feel this movement, open your mouth and take a few deep, sighing breaths. You will experience your upper chest rising and falling, a useful movement whenever there is a need for rapid, deep inhalations. But thoracic breathing (also called chest breathing) and clavicular breathing (using the neck and shoulder muscles) are the body's response to emergencies:

upright position, the upper chest becomes relatively quiet, and movement is most noticeable in the lower ribs. This has been called the "bucket-handle" action of the ribs: the lower ribs do not lift forward so much as they expand to the sides. The basic idea to remember is that natural everyday breathing in an upright position expands and contracts the lower ribs, especially to the sides, but produces only minimal movement in the upper chest. You can feel the expansion and contraction of the ribs by placing the hands along the sides of your body, midway between the navel and heart level. Round the shoulders and press the elbows forward as well. You will feel the sides of the rib cage expand as you inhale and contract as you exhale.

EXERCISE: Diaphragmatic Breathing in a Sitting Pose

▶ Sit erect in any seated posture (sitting on a flat-seated chair will do fine). Rest your hands on your thighs or in your lap. Close your eyes and gently lift your spine so that the rib cage, the abdomen, and the back are all free to expand and contract with your breathing.

▶ Soften the sides of the rib cage, and let the muscles of the abdomen and back support your posture with very modest muscle tone. Now notice how your breathing results in a quiet expansion of the lower torso. Much like a fish, whose gills expand and contract to the sides, you can feel the lateral movements of your lower ribs.

▶ The blend of movements that feels best for you is an individual matter. By observing the movement of the breath and exploring the balance of movement in the sides, front, and back, you will gradually arrive at a breath that flows easily. You will find that when it is combined with the expansion of the ribs to the sides, the abdominal movement is not nearly so pronounced as when you are lying down.

▶ Continue to observe your breathing, making it your focus. As time passes, sense the feelings of cleansing and nourishing that take place each time you breathe out and in. Let the breath become deep, smooth, and even.

▶ Now you can recognize the normal signs of diaphragmatic breathing in sitting or standing postures. You may find yourself relaxing as you continue, and

you will see in chapter 9 that this exercise naturally leads to a steady, seated practice of meditation.

STEP FOUR: STRENGTHENING THE DIAPHRAGM

Like all skeletal muscles in the human body, the diaphragm can lose muscle tone and become weak— and a weak diaphragm, usually the result of poor breathing habits, makes for inefficient breathing. A remedy for this is sandbag breathing, which gets its name because during the practice a sand-filled bag rests on the abdomen to build strength and awareness. Simple and time-effective, sandbag breathing will not only fortify the diaphragm, it will also develop relaxed control of the abdominal area, and give you the confidence you need to breathe easily.

The Seated Pose

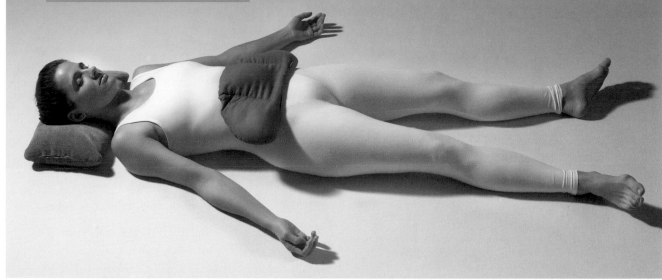

Placement of the Sandbag

EXERCISE: Sandbag Breathing

► Lie on your back with a thin cushion supporting the head and neck. The legs are slightly apart and the arms rest along the sides of the body, palms turned up. The spine is not bent to either side.

► Relax the flow of breath: feel the breath flowing out and in, over and over again; soften the abdomen and feel it rise as you inhale and fall as you exhale.

► Let the breath flow without pause between the breaths.

► Once the flow of breath is well-established, place a sandbag weighing about 10 pounds on the abdomen and begin a period of weight training. You will find that simply placing the weight on the abdomen focuses your attention there. Breathe out and in, raising the weight as you inhale and lowering the weight as you exhale. You are not pushing the bag up by deliberately protruding the abdomen; the bag rises from the contraction of the diaphragm.

► The weight on the abdomen requires you to work a little harder to inhale and expand the lungs; as you exhale, the sandbag will naturally push down, causing the breath to flow out quickly. Regulate your exhalation so that it is relaxed and approximately the same length as the inhalation. In this way sandbag breathing not only strengthens the diaphragm, it tones the muscles of the abdomen as well.

► Observe your capacity. If you become tired, take the weight off.

► Start with a practice time of about 5 minutes. Then take the weight off, relaxing the abdomen, and be aware of the new sensation. You will find a noticeable difference in the feel of your breath even after a short period of sandbag breathing. After resting for a few minutes, come back to a sitting posture.

One way to organize the practice of sandbag breathing is to establish a schedule of three days on and one day off for a month. Gradually increase the time with the sandbag from 5 minutes to 10 minutes. (Very committed students may eventually wish to place a second sandbag on top of the first, doubling the weight.) Practice once or twice a day. Be mindful of your capacity: do not increase the weight or the length of practice time too quickly. After a month you will find that your diaphragm has been strengthened, your breath will be deeper and more efficient, and you will feel noticeably more confident about your breathing. This period of a month's practice can be repeated at any time to further increase muscle tone.

Hatha yoga postures can also be used to strengthen the diaphragm. Perhaps the best for this purpose are the twisting and inverted postures. In a twisting pose the abdominal area is tightened, much like squeezing water from a dishrag by twisting it; this increases intra-abdominal pressure and forces the diaphragm to work harder as it presses against the abdominal organs. And by firmly breathing into the twisted abdomen, the diaphragm is strengthened.

To a lesser degree inverted postures can also be used for this purpose. When the body is upside down, the organs of the abdomen rest on top of the diaphragm, instead of the other way around, and the act of inhaling will require that the diaphragm lift the abdominal organs. Because the organs of the abdomen weigh a significant amount, this can also help improve muscle tone in the diaphragm.

STEP FIVE: FIVE QUALITIES OF GOOD BREATHING

The process of giving the breath a new shape requires time and experience. When we try too hard to breathe diaphragmatically, we usually manage to create new tensions. But if we do not develop a strong diaphragmatic breath we cannot relax our effort to breathe, and must unconsciously respond to breathing tensions that are largely outside our awareness. Once the breath flows easily through the nose, however, and once it can be maintained with a modest effort from the diaphragm, then attention can be given to the five basic qualities of good breathing. Good breathing is:

deep	not shallow
smooth	not jerky
even	exhalation and inhalation are of equal length
without sound	not noisy
without pause	smooth, unbroken transitions from breath to breath

Whenever you are relaxing and observing your breath you can scan for difficulties in these areas, unblocking tension and allowing the breath to unfold with the passing moments.

How Long Should I Practice?

Do not expect to change a lifetime of breathing habits overnight. Two weeks of daily practice will help you internalize the principles of diaphragmatic breathing. Six months of practice will anchor the habit and provide experience in a variety of situations that test your new breathing style. During this training period your practice of the stretches and postures found in chapters 3 and 5 will be an invaluable resource. They give you the opportunity to integrate breathing with physical movement, and to practice staying focused on breathing when the challenge of a posture might otherwise pull you away.

Training the breath can be deceptive. The mind is active. In the beginning thoughts move much more rapidly than the breath, and the speed of breathing feels painfully slow compared to that of thinking. As a result the practice may seem boring, unimportant, or tedious. Do continue with your practice, however—you will see that once the mind has adapted to the speed of breathing, it will relax.

Each day your breath training will lead you to periods of inner quiet that are not available from external sources, and soon your breath will flow almost effortlessly. The first time you experience yourself relaxing your breath in an emotionally tight spot, you will no longer wonder about the value of your work. You will have observed in action that your breath can help you survive even the most upsetting moments. And as you continue, your breathing will become steady and serene as the result of your patient efforts to deepen and relax it.

Even though

the exercises

in this chapter

can be practiced

in a number of

ways, here is a

schedule that you

may find helpful in

the beginning.

▶ Get into the habit of morning and evening practice sessions every day. These don't need to be long—perhaps 10 minutes each.

▶ Practice relaxed breath awareness in the corpse pose (p.55) for three days. Be sure to let the breath flow through the nose.

▶ Next, each morning practice breathing in the crocodile pose (p.60) and in the evening practice in the corpse pose (p.58). During this time you will become well-acquainted with the experience of diaphragmatic breathing.

▶ In addition, at the end of every session of stretching or yoga postures, lie down in the corpse pose for a period of relaxation that includes diaphragmatic breathing.

▶ After two weeks, change the morning practice. Following a brief period (2–3 minutes) in the crocodile pose, use the morning time for breath awareness in a sitting pose (p.62). Continue this for one month. During that time, gradually memorize and practice the five qualities of good breathing.

▶ If you think it would be helpful, use sandbag breathing (p.63) as a one-month substitute for the morning practice period. This can be done at any time.

▶ Finally, let your breath training evolve naturally into a regular practice of relaxation and/or meditation each morning and evening.

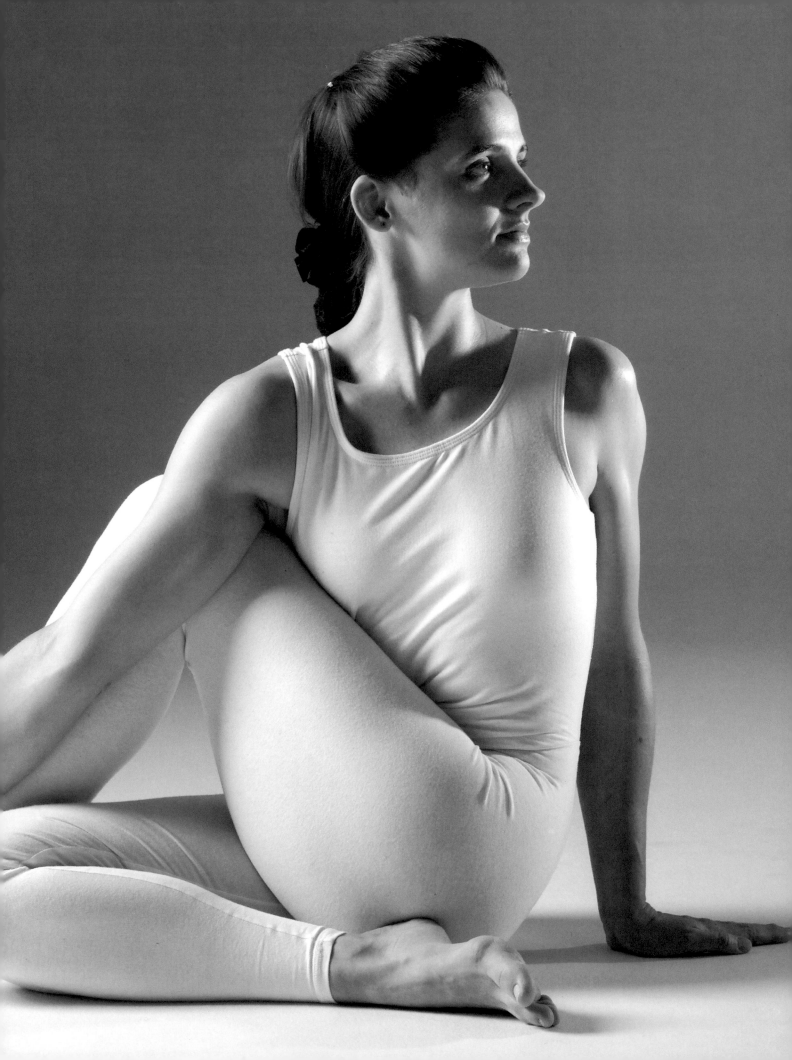

CHAPTER FIVE

ASANA SEQUENCE TWO

Make your posture steady and comfortable.
——— *Yoga Sutras of Patanjali*

deepening & strengthening

T H E sequence presented in this chapter requires more strength and skill than Asana Sequence One (chapter 3), and it incorporates more of the classic yoga postures. It also includes the sun salutation, a series of movements traditionally done at the beginning of asana practice. You will want to be comfortable with the first sequence before replacing it with this one (it may take a number of months of regular practice, or longer, before you're ready). Asana Sequence One will give you a good understanding of your body and gradually improve your flexibility, strength, and balance. Asana Sequence Two will allow your asana practice to unfold.

The challenge here is not only to train muscles and joints but also to refine awareness of your body, and to incorporate breath awareness and the qualities of good breathing into the poses. Sustained breath awareness is a conscious element of each pose, and each movement in and out of a posture can be linked with the breath. The importance of this cannot be overstated, for it is the coordination of body, breath, and mind that balances the nervous system and unlocks the power of hatha yoga.

Unbroken breath awareness not only trains the mind, it integrates the energy of each posture and directs it along to the next one. The following sequence of poses works because of this flow of awareness. Think of your postures not as isolated, independent events, but as a smooth progression of dynamic positions that build on and complement each other. Each pose allows you to release the challenges and tensions of the previous postures and prepares you for the ones that follow.

The movements in this chapter are more complex than those in chapter 3, so before attempting a pose read through the entire description and examine the accompanying photographs. You can perform some postures in stages, one step at a time, which will allow you to process each instruction as you progress through the pose. But other postures require that you keep the steps flowing without interruption to prevent muscle fatigue and strain, so you will need to remember and internalize the instructions. In either case, repetition is the key that will allow you to gradually internalize the instructions and make the poses your own. For your convenience, the entire sequence is illustrated at the end of the chapter.

Asana Sequence Two

PRELIMINARY PRACTICES

Before attempting the poses in this sequence it is important to first center the mind and stretch the body. Centering can be accomplished standing in the mountain pose, or resting on the floor in the corpse or crocodile pose. Then, after centering, you can warm up with the short selection of stretches from Sequence One listed on the next page. The selection can be varied and even lengthened if necessary to address areas of your body that feel particularly tight or restricted. But at the least, stretch overhead; move the shoulders and arms; bend forward, backward, and to the side; twist the body; and do the abdominal squeeze 5 times. Complete your warming up with the sun salutation.

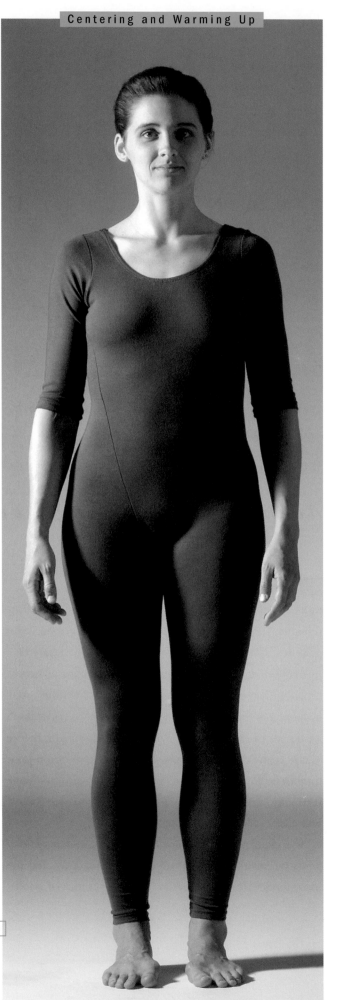

Centering and Warming Up

The Mountain Pose

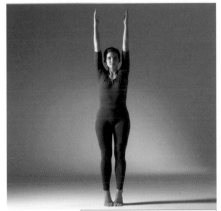

Overhead Stretch

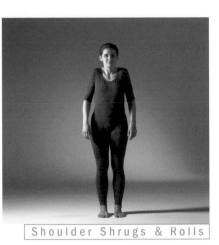

Shoulder Shrugs & Rolls

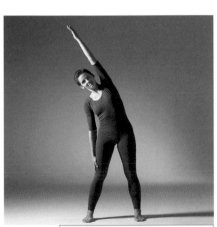

Arm Circles

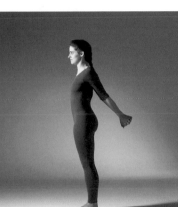

Chest Expander

1

Centering and Warming Up

Stand in the mountain pose. Let your eyes close, sense the contact of your feet against the floor, and lengthen upward through the crown of the head. Be aware of your breathing, feeling the breath cleanse as it flows out and nourish as it flows in. Let your posture become steady and balanced.

Now begin the short sequence of warm-up stretches selected from Asana Sequence One (chapter 3) and pictured here. Repeat each stretch until you feel prepared to move on.

Standing Side Bend

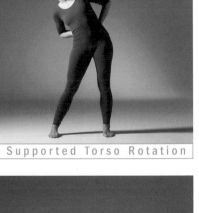

Supported Torso Rotation

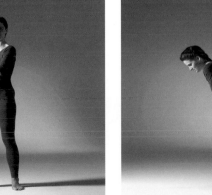

Standing Warm-Up Twist

Abdominal Squeeze

SUN SALUTATION (SURYA NAMASKARA)

The sun salutation is a sequence of 12 classic postures that traditionally begins every asana practice session. There is no better remedy for sluggishness, erratic energy, stiffness, or a bad mood than the sun salutation. It stretches and strengthens all the major muscle groups, flexes the spine forward and backward, activates the navel center (solar plexus), stimulates circulation, and warms the body. It coordinates body, mind, and breath, and awakens a sense of joy.

Sun Salutation Sequence

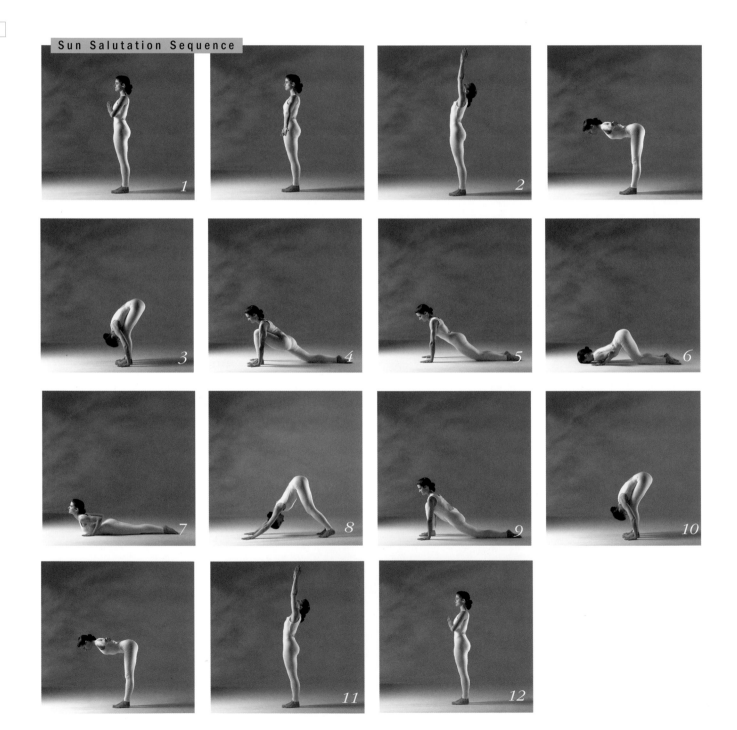

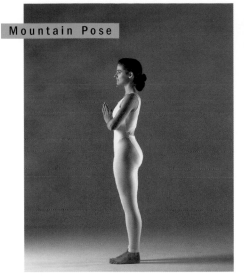

Mountain Pose

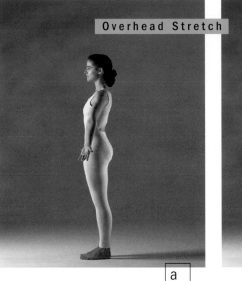

Overhead Stretch

a

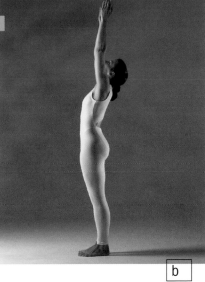

b

STEPS OF THE
SUN SALUTATION

Step One

Step Two

Mountain Pose with Hands at the Chest (Tadasana)

Stand with the feet hip-width apart and parallel, your weight centered over the arches of the feet. Press down through the feet as you lift and lengthen the spine through the top of the head. Bring the palms together at the heart in a gesture of inwardness and respect. Then widen and slightly elevate the chest, moving the shoulders down and away from the ears. Close the eyes and focus on the flow of the breath.

Overhead Stretch

a) Open the eyes and release the arms to the sides. Inhaling, slowly sweep the arms out to the sides and overhead, turning the palms at shoulder level and continuing up until the palms face each other. (This arm variation reduces strain on the back.)

b) As you raise the arms, lift the chest and look up, keeping the back of the neck long. Keep the arms straight and the palms pressed together or facing each other.

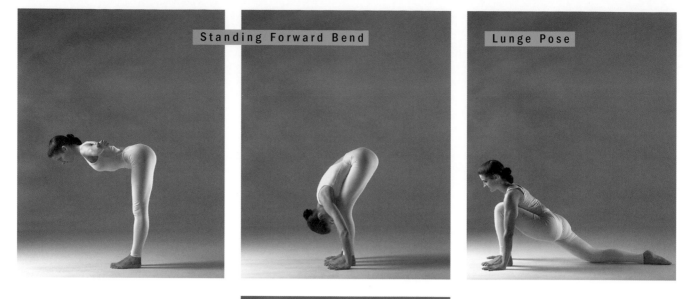

Standing Forward Bend

Lunge Pose

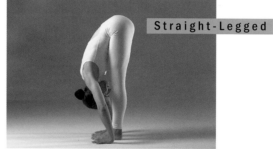

Straight-Legged

Step Three

Step Four

Standing Forward Bend

a) With an exhalation, lengthen the spine and bend forward from the hips as you lower the arms out to the side. Keep the back straight and the shoulders pulled down away from the ears.

b) Bend the knees when you feel the back starting to round, and place the hands on the floor beside the feet. Lengthen the spine as you release the head, shoulders, and arms toward the floor. Lift the sitting bones by contracting the abdominal muscles, drawing the abdomen toward the thighs. If you are comfortable, you may perform this step with straight legs.

Lunge Pose

On an inhalation, step back with the right leg, lowering the knee and the top of the foot to the floor. The left knee is directly above the left ankle, the shin perpendicular. The fingers stay in line with the toes. Allow the pelvis to settle toward the floor, lengthening the front of the body as the pelvis descends. Breathe into the abdomen, softening resistance.

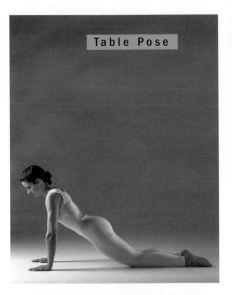

Table Pose

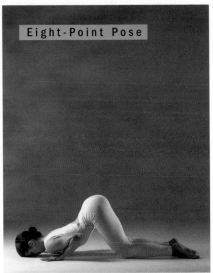

Eight-Point Pose

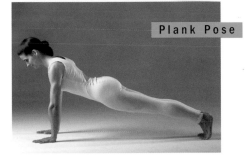

Plank Pose

Step Five

Step Six

Table Pose

Without moving your hands or right knee, bring the left knee in line with the right so your knees are hip-width apart and you are on your hands and knees. Draw the shoulder blades down and lengthen from the base of the spine through the top of the head.

Downward-Facing Plank Pose

When you are ready, you may substitute the downward-facing plank pose for the table pose. To come into the downward-facing plank from the lunge pose, turn the toes of the right foot under, lift the knee, and press the heel away. Without lifting the pelvis, bring the left leg back alongside the right. The body is straight and firm from the top of the head to the heels. Make sure the pelvis remains in line.

Eight-Point Pose

Exhale and lower the knees, chest, and forehead (or chin) to the floor. Keep the spine arched, the pelvis up, and the arms close to the sides.

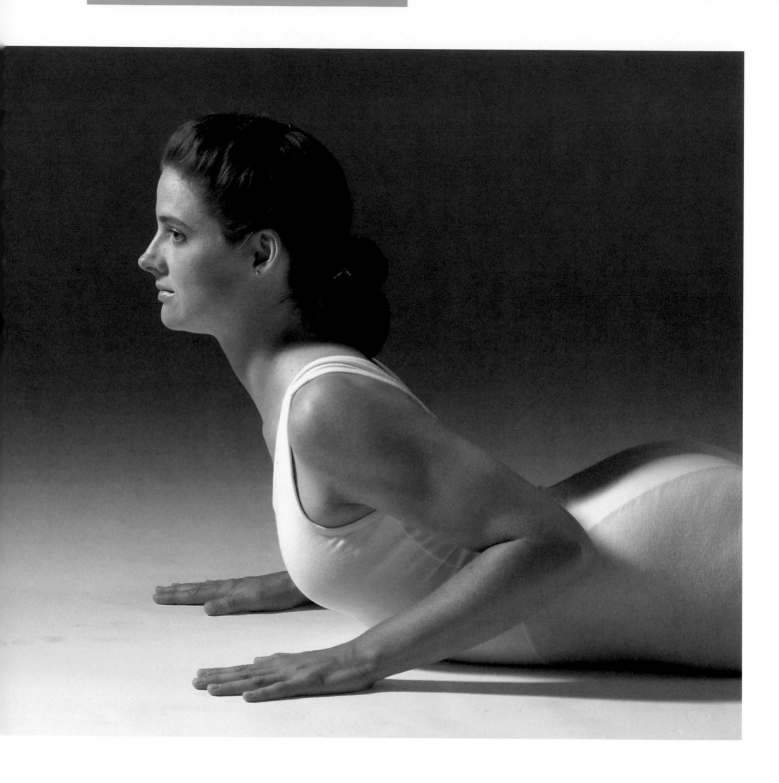

Unsupported Cobra Pose

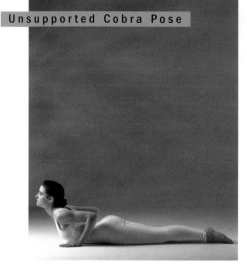

Downward-Facing Dog Pose

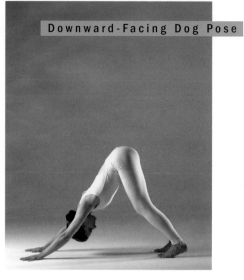

Straight-Legged

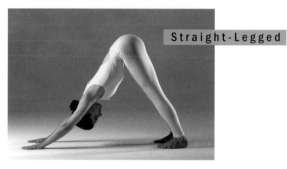

Step Seven

Step Eight

Unsupported Cobra Pose

On an inhalation lower the pelvis
and release the body to the floor,
lengthening the spine. Keep the
palms on the floor next to the chest
with the fingers pointing forward
and the arms hugging the sides of
the ribs. Keeping the buttocks and
legs firm, press the pelvis into the
floor and draw the shoulder blades
together and down the back. Now
inhale and slide the nose forward,
using the muscles of the back to
lift the head and chest. Keep the
shoulders pulled back and down,
and the elbows in. Do not push
with the hands.

Downward-Facing Dog Pose

Next, exhale and press the hands down into the floor, turn the toes under,
and lift the pelvis up and back. Keep the knees bent, and remain on the
balls of your feet as you flatten your back and raise the sitting bones.
Lengthen the spine and widen between the shoulder blades. Let the neck be
a relaxed extension of the spine. To deepen the stretch, gradually straighten
the legs and lower the heels toward the floor. Do not round the back or lose
the lift in the sitting bones. Hold for 1–3 breaths.

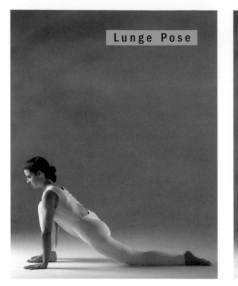

Lunge Pose

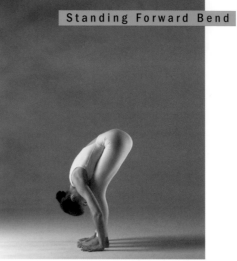

Standing Forward Bend

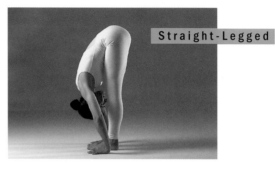

Straight-Legged

Step Nine

Step Ten

Lunge Pose

From the downward-facing dog pose, inhale and step forward with the right foot, placing it between the hands with toes in line with the fingertips. As you bring the leg forward, a slight shift in your weight toward the left will help create space for the movement of the right leg. Place the left knee and the top of the left foot on the floor and extend the leg. Align the right knee over the ankle. Allow the pelvis to settle toward the floor, lengthening the front of the body as the pelvis descends. Feel the breath in the abdomen, softening resistance.

Standing Forward Bend

Now, turn the toes of the left foot under. With an exhalation shift the weight onto the right leg. Lift the pelvis and step forward with the left foot, bringing it alongside the right (move the leg in stages if necessary). Straighten both legs, elevating the sitting bones—but keep the knees bent if necessary to keep the spine long or to protect the back. Keep your hands alongside the feet and release the head toward the floor.

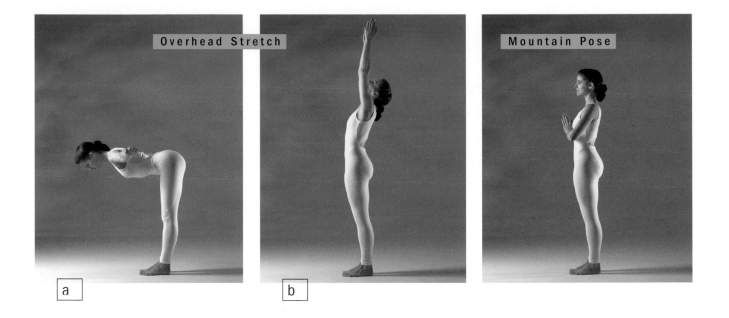

Overhead Stretch   a   b   Mountain Pose

Overhead Stretch

a) With an inhalation, bend the knees, and open the arms out to the side as you lengthen the spine parallel to the floor. Lift the torso, keeping the spine straight as you come up.

b) Stretch the arms overhead and lift the chest, looking up between the hands.

Mountain Pose

As you exhale, sweep the arms out to the side and down. Then once more bring the palms together at the chest. Pause and relax, aware of the flow of the breath as the body becomes quiet. Then repeat the 12 steps, this time initiating the backward and forward steps with the left leg instead of the right. In this way the sun salutation is practiced in sets of two. Begin with 1–3 sets. When you are finished, stand quietly in the mountain pose until your breath is calm and tranquil.

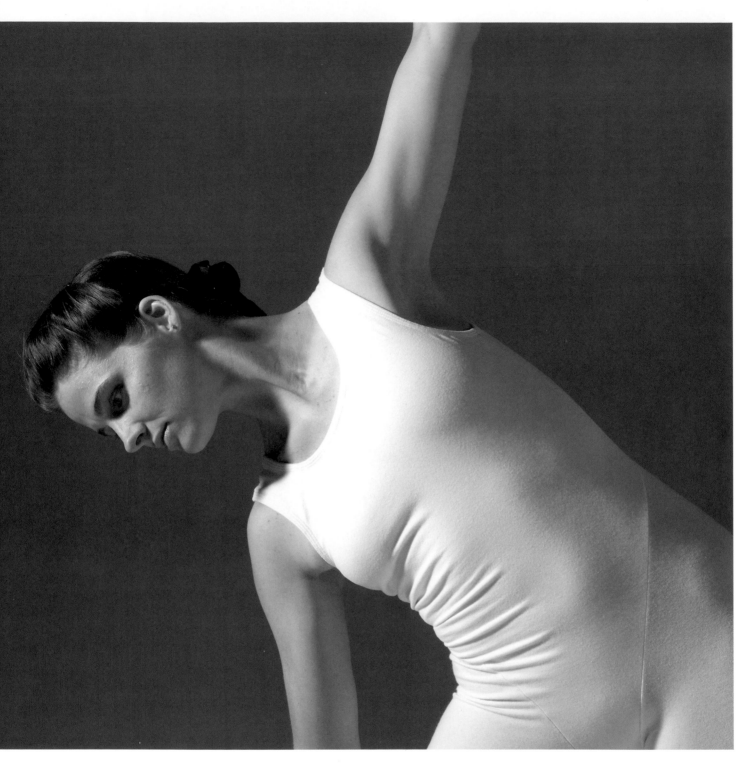

STANDING POSES

The standing poses develop both strength and flexibility; they provide the foundation for other postures. They are important poses not only in the beginning stages of practice when we need balance and integrated awareness, but also as we begin to improve the way we sit, stand, walk, and use the body in daily life.

The standing poses improve circulation, digestion, and elimination, and give us confidence, willpower, stamina, and stability.

In all standing poses pay attention to the alignment of the feet, knees, and pelvis. Keep the joints, especially the knees, firm, but not locked, and when working with a bent knee, keep the knee directly in line with the foot.

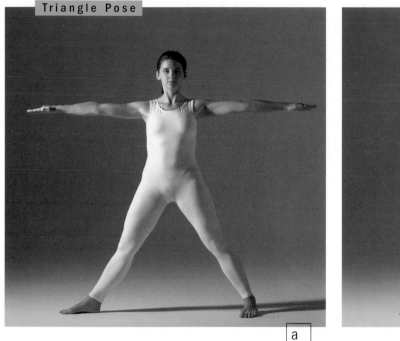

Triangle Pose

a

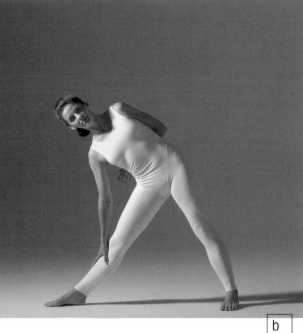

b

3

Triangle Pose (Trikonasana)

a) From the mountain pose, bring the feet 3–4 feet (or a leg's length) apart. Pivot the right foot 90 degrees to the right, and turn the left foot in slightly by moving the heel away. The heel of the right foot should be in line with the arch of the left foot, and both soles should rest firmly on the floor. Keep the pelvis level and facing forward, sensing a feeling of openness through the front of the pelvis and thighs which extends throughout the body. Then in one smooth movement, inhale and raise the arms directly out to the sides, keeping the shoulders down and broadening from the center of the chest. Relax and breathe.

b) Now lower the left arm and place the forearm on the lower back. Exhaling, shift the pelvis to the left and move the shoulders to the right, bringing the right shoulder out and over the leg. Smoothly continue the movement, bending to the right (bend from the top of the leg, not the waist) and placing the right hand on the leg either slightly above or just below the knee. The weight of the body is only partially supported by the arm.

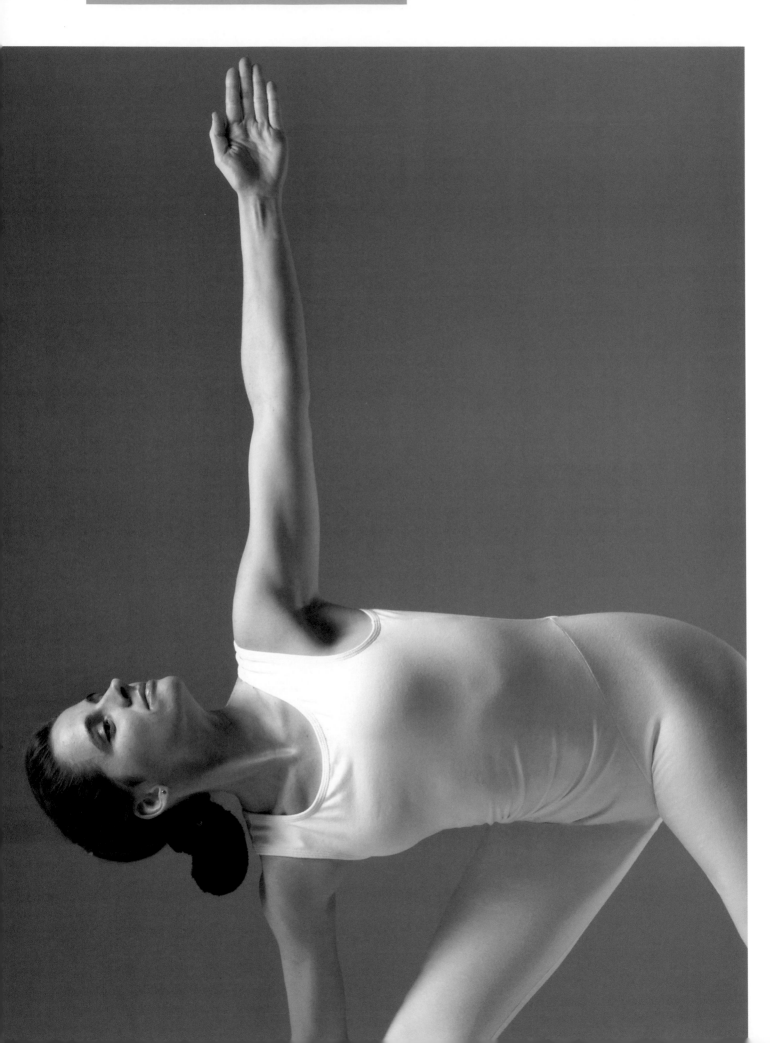

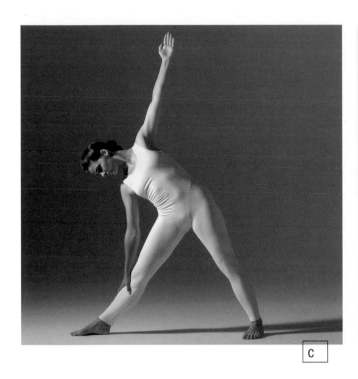

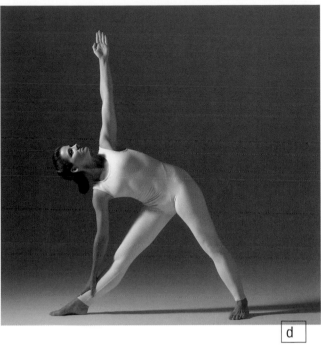

c) Turn the head to look at the right foot, aligning the neck with the leg. While maintaining this alignment on the right side of the body, shift your awareness to the left side. Widen the pelvis by drawing the left hip back. Then move your attention upward, opening the abdomen, chest, and shoulder. Keep both thighs active, further widening the pelvis. Finally, raise the arm and extend it from the shoulder, palm facing forward. Relax in the pose, breathing and sensing the expansion of the entire front of the body.

You may wish to complete the posture here. If you are ready to come out, exhale, press through the ball of the right foot and lift, keeping the spine long. If you are a bit shaky, bending the right knee makes it easier to lift out of the pose. Reestablish balance with a few relaxed breaths, and repeat this much of the pose on the other side.

▶Benefits: Stretches the spine and spinal nerves laterally; increases flexibility in the hip joints; adjusts the sacrum and lower back; stretches the back of the legs. Integrates body awareness; develops both strength and flexibility; improves structural alignment.

d) To deepen the downward movement, broaden from the center of the chest, and lengthen through the left arm as well as through the back of the right leg. Elongate the spine and move the hand down the leg, relaxing resistance in the left side and in the right hamstrings, and allowing the weight of the upper arm to help you lower further. Rest the right hand at the ankle (or if you are flexible enough, grasp the big toe or place the hand on the floor outside the foot). To gain these deeper stretches, however, do not rotate the left hip forward, sacrificing the expansion you have achieved in the pelvis and torso. You may look down at the foot, straight ahead, or up toward the extended arm. Relax and breathe as you hold the pose.

When you are ready to come out, exhale, press through the ball of the right foot and lift, keeping the spine long. If you feel unstable, bending the right knee makes it easier to lift out of the pose. Finally, turn your feet to the center, reestablish balance with a few relaxed breaths, and repeat the triangle pose on the other side.

Angle Pose

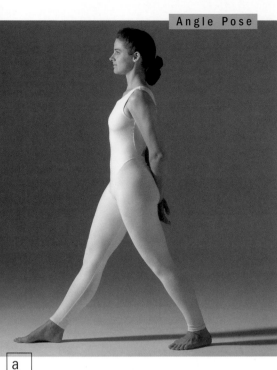

a

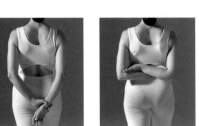

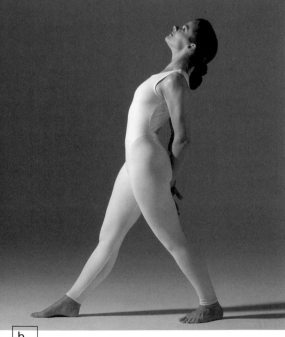

b

Angle Pose (Parshvottanasana)

a) Stand with your feet about 3 feet apart. Pivot the right foot 90 degrees to the right, and angle the left foot in slightly more than in the triangle pose. Rotate the pelvis and torso to face the right leg. Bring the arms behind the back and either hold the right wrist with the left hand or hold the opposite elbows.

b) Rotate the pelvis further to the right by bringing the left hip forward and the right hip back. Then ground the feet, and lengthen upward through the legs and pelvis. Elongate the spine, lift the chest, and gaze slightly upward.

c) On an exhalation slowly bend forward from the hips until the upper body is parallel to the floor. As you bend forward the sitting bones are lifted, stretching the hamstrings. Keep the lower back flat and the pelvis level.

You may wish to complete the pose here. If you are ready to come out, inhale, press through the ball of the right foot and lift, keeping the spine long. Bending the right knee makes it easier to lift out of the pose. Reestablish balance with a few relaxed breaths, and repeat this much of the pose on the other side.

d) To bend further, elongate the spine, draw the right kneecap up, and relax resistance in the hamstrings. To maintain balance as you lower, place your hands on your leg or on the floor on either side of your foot (or, you may keep the arms behind the back).

e) Then lengthen and draw the abdomen, chest, and face down toward the leg. Relax the back of the neck, remaining centered over the leg. Watch the breath, relaxing resistance.

When you are ready to come out, clasp the hands behind the back, inhale, press through the ball of the right foot and lift, keeping the spine long. Bending the right knee makes it easier to lift out of the pose. Finally, turn your feet to the center, reestablish balance with a few relaxed breaths, and repeat the angle pose on the other side.

▶Benefits: Stretches the hamstrings; builds strength and flexibility in the legs and pelvis; stretches the hip rotators in the pelvis (felt deep in the buttocks); improves balance.

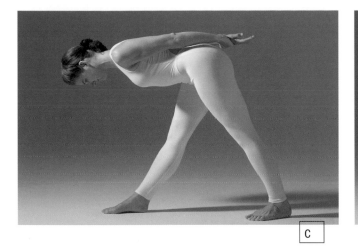

c

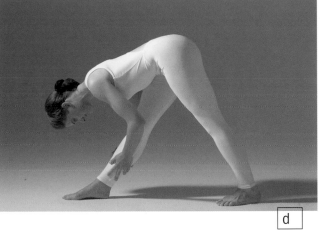

d

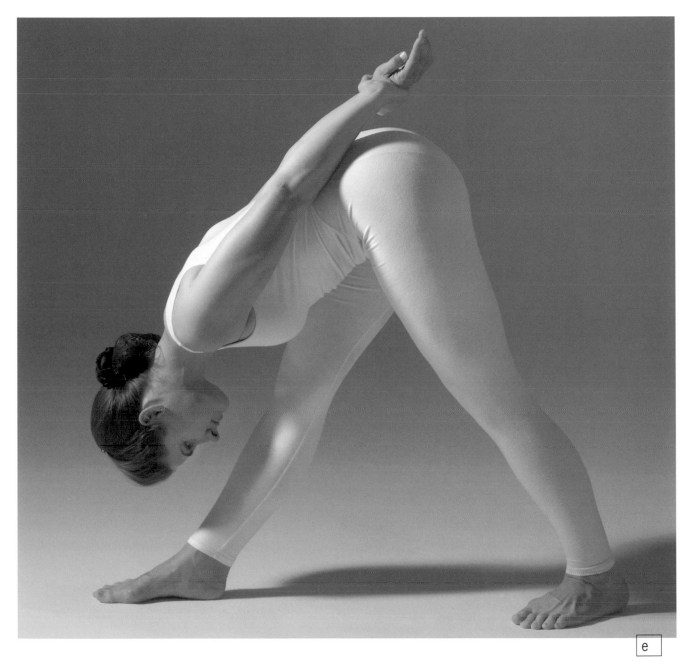

e

Standing Spread-Legged Forward Bend

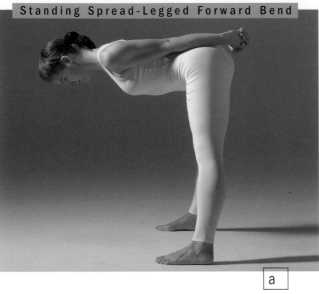

a

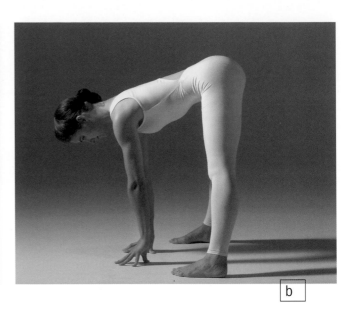

b

5

**Standing Spread-Legged Forward Bend
(Prasarita Padottanasana)**

a) Stand with the feet 3–4 feet apart and parallel. Clasp the hands behind the back and open the chest and shoulders. Exhaling, slowly bend forward from the hips. As you stretch out and down, keep your weight evenly balanced on your feet. Keep the back flat and broaden through the shoulders and neck.

b) Without pausing in the movement, release the hands and place the fingertips on the floor below the shoulders, keeping the arms straight. If you cannot reach the floor, place a support beneath your hands, or bend the knees to keep the spine long and the hands on the floor. Look down at the floor, lengthening the neck. As you relax and breathe, tilt the pelvis forward, drawing the pubic bones between the thighs. This powerful movement not only flattens the lower back, it also lifts and widens the sitting bones and spreads the insides of the thighs. (With experience you will find that the pelvis tilts and the sitting bones spread naturally as you come down into the pose.) Hold the pose and breathe.

c) Next, center the right hand on the floor. Exhale and twist the torso, smoothly sweeping the left arm out and up. Expand from the center of the chest out through the fingertips. Lengthen the neck, turn the head, and look toward the left hand. Inhaling, twist back to the center and repeat the movement with the breath 3–5 times. On the last repetition, hold the extension for 3–5 breaths. Then release and change sides.

d) To deepen the forward bend, place the hands on the floor under the shoulders. Bend your elbows as you draw the abdomen between the legs, lowering the top of the head toward the floor. Keep the lower back flat and bend from the hip joints.

e) Or you may clasp the hands behind you and then raise the arms and bring them over the back of the head toward the floor, letting the weight of the arms assist in bringing you further down. Hold and breathe, relaxing in the pose.

To come out of the pose, return the arms to the back. With an inhalation, flatten the lower back and gracefully lengthen and lift the head, neck, and upper back, bending the knees as necessary to keep the lower back strong and the spine long. Release your hands, step your feet together, and relax in the mountain pose, watching the flow of the breath.

▶Benefits: This series stretches the hamstring muscles and adductor muscles of the thighs; increases flexibility at the hip joints; strengthens deep lower back and pelvic muscles; twists and stretches the entire torso; improves balance.

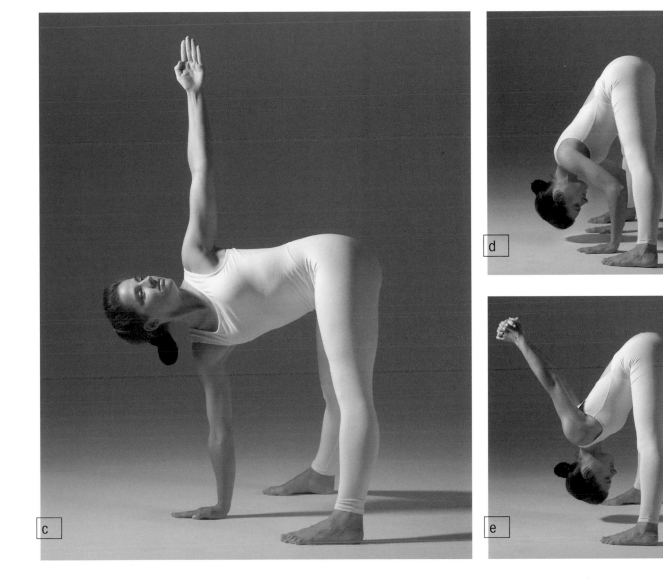

6

Tree Pose (Vrikshasana)

a) Begin in the mountain pose with the feet together and parallel. Center the pelvis over the feet, and lengthen the spine up out of the pelvis. Focus your eyes on a point on the floor or on the wall in front of you. Then bring the sole of the left foot to the right inner ankle as you open the left hip and rotate the knee out to the side. For easier balance keep the toes touching the floor. Press the palms together at the center of the chest, and lengthen through the top of the head.

b) When you are ready to move on, lift the left foot and press the sole against the calf or inner thigh. Raise the arms overhead (either by sweeping them out to the sides or by lifting them directly up). The palms may either touch or face one another. Stretch up through the torso, lifting the chest, and extending up through the crown of the head. Steady your balance and follow the flow of the breath for as long as you enjoy the pose. To come out, exhale and lower the arms and foot back to the mountain pose. Stand quietly with your attention on the breath. Then repeat on the other side.

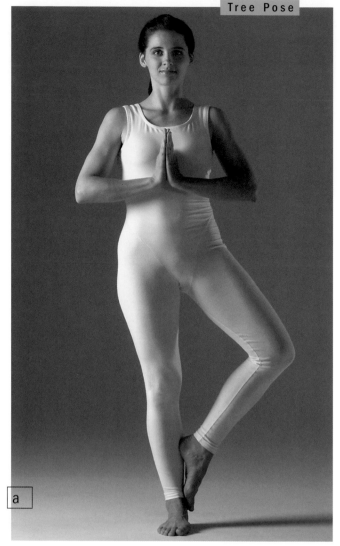

Tree Pose

a

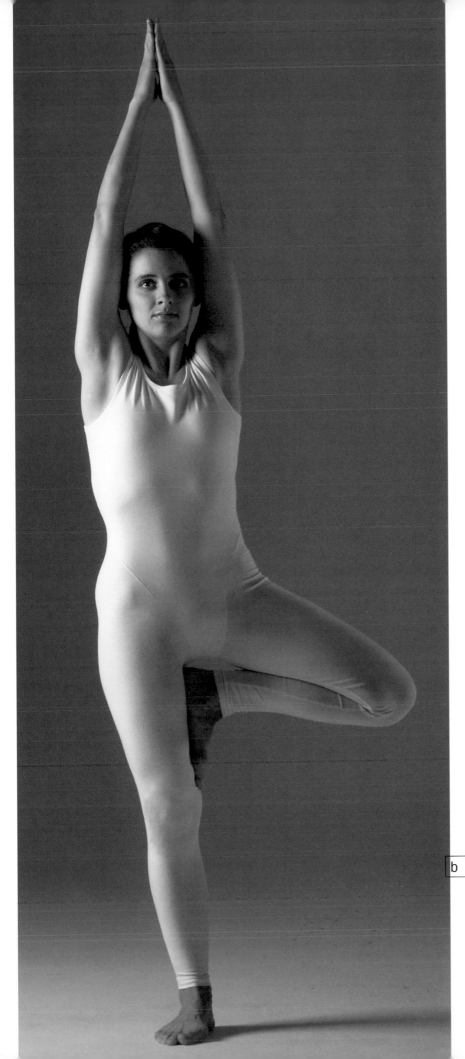

▶Benefits: Improves balance and
concentration; strengthens the
muscles of the legs and pelvis;
opens the chest and shoulders;
improves the quality of the breath.

b

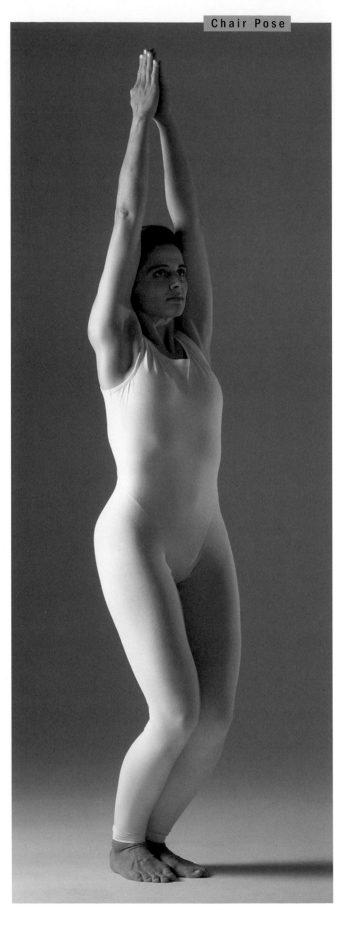

Chair Pose (Utkatasana)

Stand with the feet together. Inhaling, raise the arms
to the sides and overhead. Extend the arms straight up
and alongside the ears. Press the palms together without
bending the elbows, or stretch up through the fingers
with the palms facing. Now exhale as you bend the
knees, and lower the hips toward the floor, pressing the
knees together. Keep the feet flat on the floor and avoid
rounding the back. Squeeze the thighs together and
draw the pelvic floor inward and upward. Gaze forward
and breathe evenly without pause while maintaining
the upward extension of the spine and arms. Sense the
vibrancy of this pose and let the flow of energy you
experience strengthen the vertical alignment. When you
are ready, straighten the legs and exhale as you lower
the arms.

▶Benefits: At first glimpse, the effects of this pose seem
obvious: it develops strength in the muscles of the legs
and torso, and flexibility in the ankles and shoulders.
However, the pose has deeper effects. As muscles of
the inner thighs and pelvic floor contract, energy is
drawn upward. Lowering more deeply into the posture
shifts the focus of the pelvic contraction from back to
front, gradually resulting in increased strength and
muscular coordination in the entire region. Then the
vitality of the posture is ignited and the mind is focused
along the vertical lines of energy within the body.

After the strenuous standing poses, these postures rest the body and refresh the legs. They also open the lower back and spine, reestablish deep relaxed breathing, and gently awaken the navel center, which is the seat of vitality, energy, courage, and enthusiasm. Strong, flexible abdominal muscles coupled with proper breathing are essential for vibrant good health, as well as for progressing in asana practice. Be particularly mindful of the breath as you work with the poses in this section.

Child's Pose

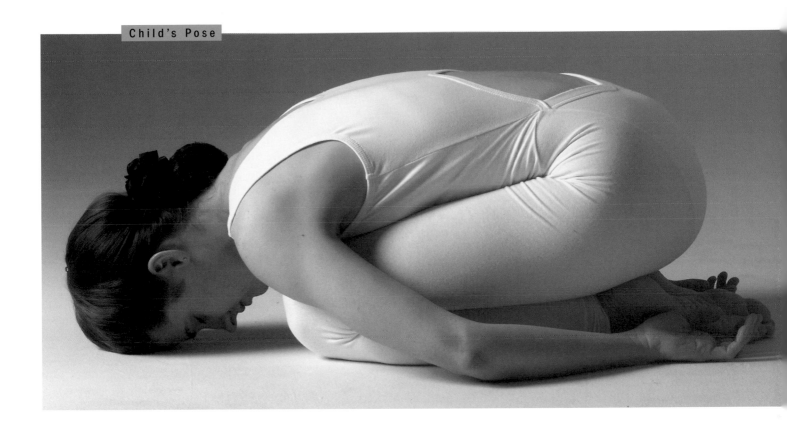

8

Child's Pose (Balasana)

Sit in a kneeling position with the tops of the feet on the floor and the buttocks resting on the heels. With an erect spine, exhale and bend forward from the hips, folding the abdomen to the thighs. Lower the forehead to the floor and rest the arms alongside the body, palms turned up. Feel the motion of the breath against the thighs and at the sides of the rib cage. Relax until the breath is steady and smooth and the mind is ready to continue. If the posture is uncomfortable you may need to spread the knees slightly or place cushions under the ankles or the back of the thighs. An alternative is to lie on the back, bringing the knees to the chest. To come out of this pose and into the next one, lift the head, flatten the back, and return to an upright posture.

▶Benefits: Relieves lower back tension; gently stretches the spine; massages the abdominal organs; refreshes the legs; quiets the mind.

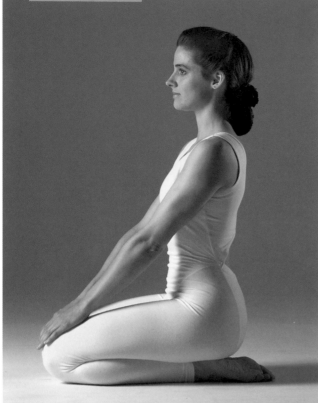

Kneeling Pose

9

Kneeling Pose (Vajrasana)

Sit on the heels with the tops of the feet on the floor. Gently press the palms onto the thighs. With the lower back erect, lift the chest and lengthen the spine up from the tailbone through the crown of the head. Close the eyes and follow the flow of the breath, momentarily deepening into the stillness of the pose. If the knees or ankles are uncomfortable, sit in a simple cross-legged pose instead.

Caution: Do not practice this pose if you experience pain in the knees.

▶Benefits: Relaxes the body; stretches the feet, ankles, and knees; refreshes the legs; restores natural breathing; develops good spinal alignment; prepares the mind to continue with the sequence.

10

**Beginning Fire Series
(Single Leglifts and Bicycling)**

a) Sit on the floor with the legs extended straight out in front of you. Lean back on the forearms with the elbows under the shoulders. Lift the chest and keep the chin toward the throat. Bend the right knee and press the foot flat on the floor near the pelvis. Now inhale and lift the left leg to the vertical, keeping the leg straight and stretching the toes toward the ceiling. Exhale and lower the leg, touching the floor but without releasing the weight. Then inhale and again lift the straight leg. Keep the jaw and face relaxed, and focus on the navel center. Move smoothly with the breath 5 times. Then change sides and repeat 5 times on the other side.

b) For a more challenging exercise, start with both legs straight out in front of you. Inhale and lift one leg, keeping the opposite leg on the floor. Exhale and lower the leg. Inhale and lift the opposite leg. Repeat 5 times, alternating sides.

Or you may in a vertical scissors-like movement begin lifting the second leg as you start to lower the first. The legs will pass in midair, and will not quite touch the floor on the downward movement. Keep the movements smooth and do not hold the breath.

c) Bicycle Leglifts. Start with both legs straight out in front of you. Bend one knee and draw the thigh toward the chest. Now reverse legs, alternately pushing and pulling like a piston. Keep the extended leg parallel to the floor and a few inches above it. Push out through the heel of the extended leg as you pull the bent leg in. Complete 5 cycles.

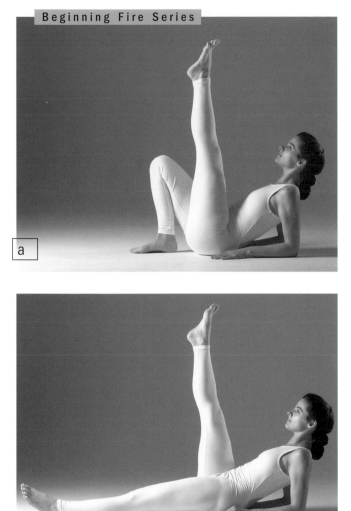

a

b

Caution: If you experience unusual pain or discomfort in the back, neck, or shoulders during or after these exercises, consult with a teacher before continuing.

▶ <u>Benefits</u>: Strengthens the abdominal muscles; increases vitality; improves digestion, elimination, and circulation.

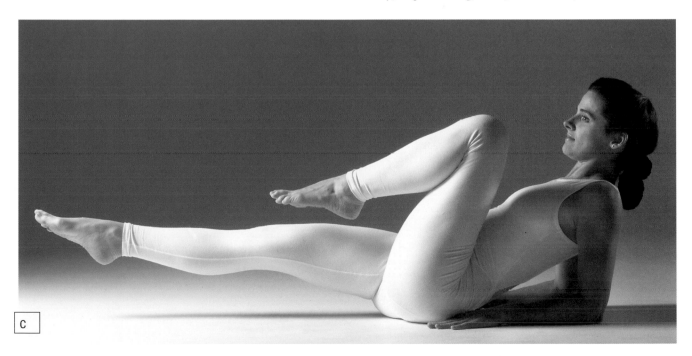

c

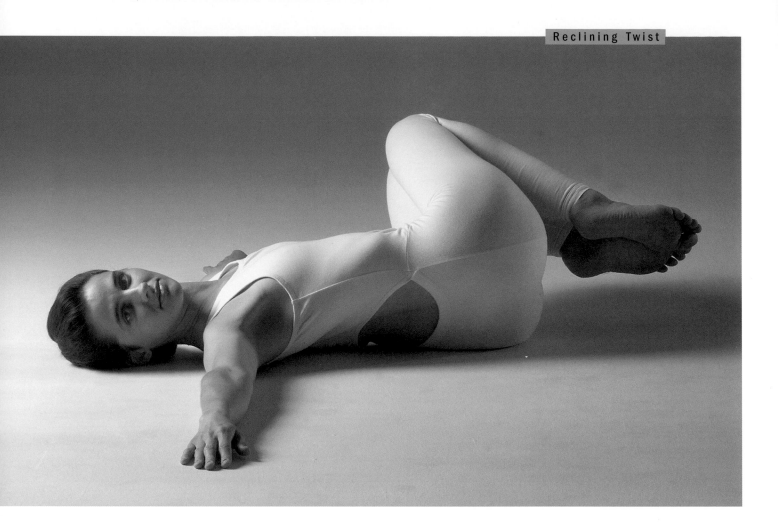

11

Reclining Twist

Lie on your back and stretch the arms directly out to the sides, palms down. Bend the knees, and bring the thighs toward the abdomen, keeping the legs together. Now gently twist from side to side, lowering the legs toward the floor. Keep the upper back and shoulders on the floor, and the legs together. Soften the lower back as you roll across it to give a massaging action to the pose. Repeat 5–10 times, then rest with the feet on the floor near the pelvis. Close your eyes and relax, feeling the flow of the breath in the pelvis, lower back, and abdomen.

▶ Benefits: Strengthens the abdominal muscles while increasing flexibility and releasing tension in the lower and mid-spine.

BACKWARD BENDS

The backward bends are among the most stimulating and energizing postures. They are powerful antidotes to sluggishness, poor breathing habits, and a host of physical ills, and they counter the tendency most of us have to collapse forward in our daily activities. The key to successful backward bends is to extend evenly through the spine, and to avoid overbending or compressing the lower back or the back of the neck. Try to create space in the entire length of the spine. In performing backward bends, keep the spine elongated, the buttocks contracted, the pelvis tucked, and the chest lifted.

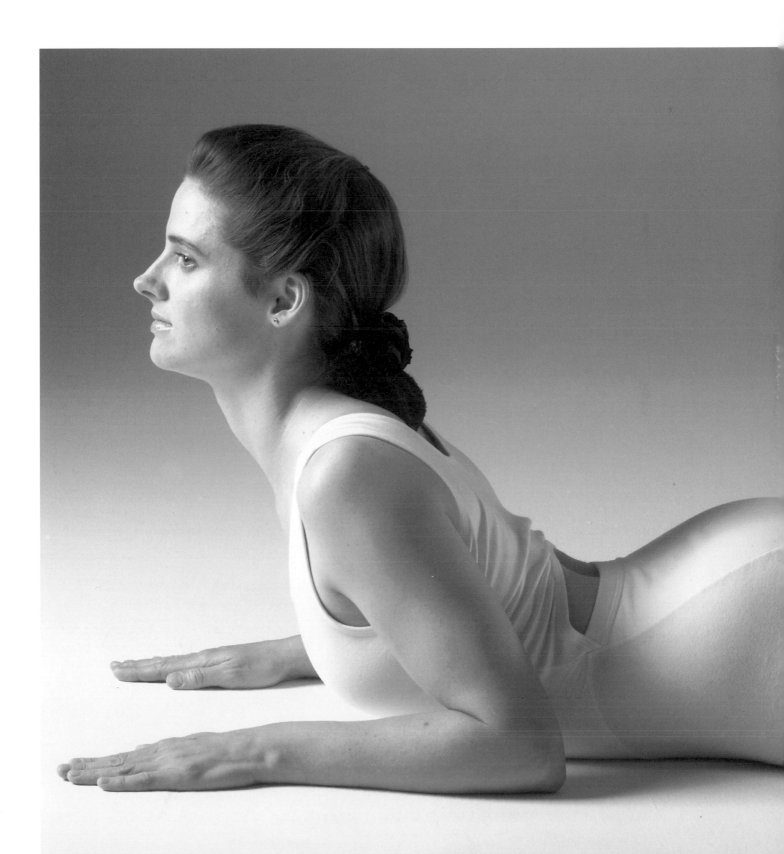

Unsupported Cobra Pose (Bhujangasana)

a) Lie on the floor face down, legs and feet together. Place the palms on the floor next to the chest or under the shoulders (the further back the hands, the more intense the pose). The fingers point forward and the arms hug the sides of the ribs. Keeping the buttocks and legs firm, press the pelvis into the floor and draw the shoulder blades together and down the back.

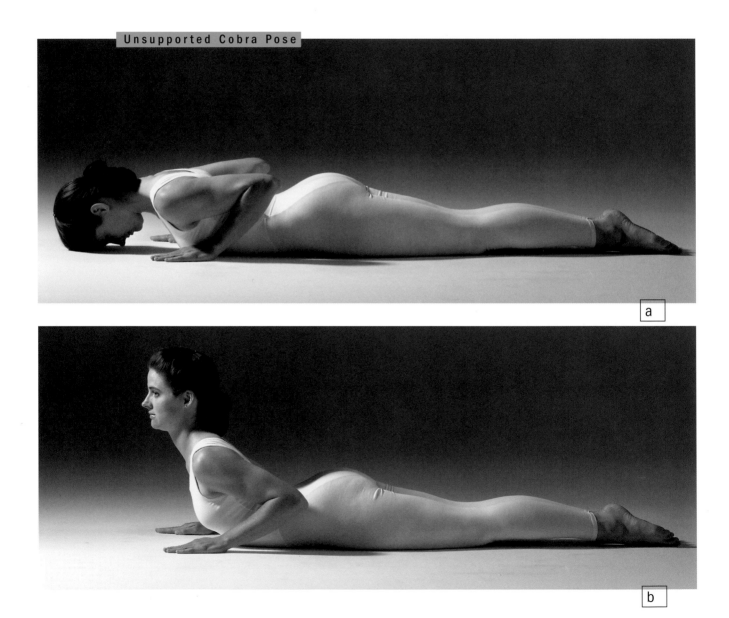

Unsupported Cobra Pose

a

b

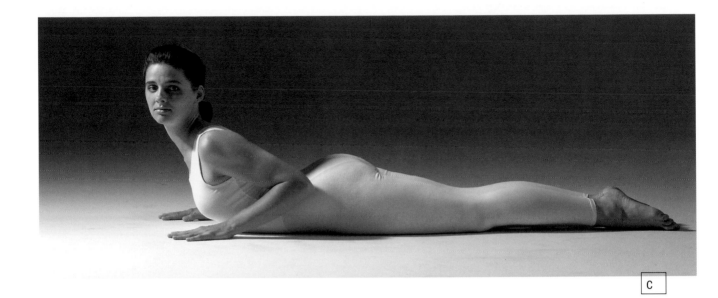

C

b) Inhale and slide the nose forward as you lift the head and chest. Keep the shoulders pulled back and down, and the elbows in. Observe the breath at the abdomen and along the sides of the lower rib cage as you center in the pose. Lengthen the spine and lift the chest with each inhalation. Exhaling, maintain the arch of the spine.

Note: There should be no weight on the hands. Do not push into the posture by pressing your hands into the floor. Strong arms can force the back into a position of strain.

Maintain the pose for 5 breaths, then exhale down, extending and lowering the chin to the floor first, then the nose, and finally the forehead. Turn the head to one side and rest for a few breaths. Then repeat the pose and turn the head to the opposite side when coming out the second time.

c) To increase mobility in the neck and shoulders, come into the pose for a third time. Turn the head slowly from side to side (as if to look behind you), while keeping the shoulders down. Then return the chin to the center for a few breaths. Release out of the pose as before by exhaling and lowering the sternum, chin, nose, and forehead to the floor. Bring the arms down alongside the body and turn the head to the side, resting and watching the flow of the breath. Repeat 2–3 times.

▶Benefits: Strengthens the muscles of the back; improves circulation to the intervertebral discs; opens the throat, chest, and abdomen; improves mobility and alignment of the spine; helps with low back pain; facilitates proper breathing patterns.

Locust Pose (Shalabhasana)

a) Single-Leg Locust Pose. Lie on your stomach with the chin on the floor and the legs together: the arms are alongside, with the palms facing the body. Close the hands in a loose fist. Keep the feet together and point the toes, elongating the entire body. Contract the buttocks and press the abdomen into the floor.

Inhale, extend the right leg through the toes, and lift the leg 8–14 inches without bending the knee. Lift firmly with the right buttock

and lower back, and avoid pressing the left knee into the floor to assist the movement. The knees and tops of the feet face downward. No matter how high you lift, keep both sides of the pelvis on the floor, and the chin down. Hold the pose for several breaths and then repeat on the other side. Practice this version of the posture until you develop sufficient strength to do the following double-leg version comfortably.

b) Double-Leg Locust Pose. Lie on your stomach as before, with the legs together and the arms alongside the body. Slide the arms under the body so that the forearms lie on the inner side of the front edge of the hipbone. Make fists and rest the upper thigh or groin on the little-finger side of the fists, pressing the thumb side into the floor. Keep the arms straight, and draw the elbows together. Inhaling, press the

Locust Pose

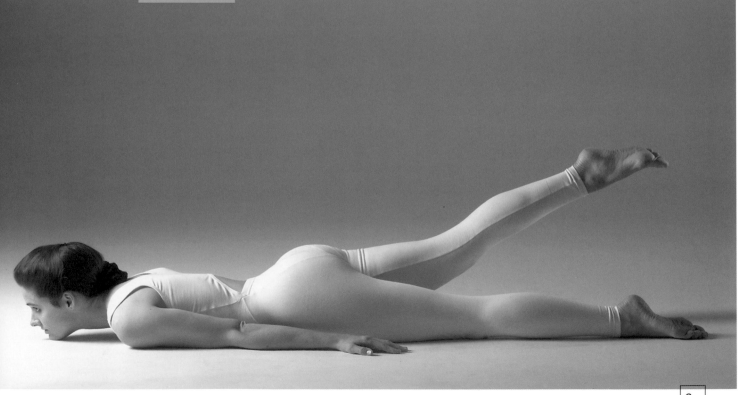

a

arms into the floor and raise both legs. Continue to breathe. Keep the legs no more than hip-width apart, and point the toes to help stretch the legs up and back. Hold briefly, then release slowly back to the floor.

▶Benefits: Strengthens the legs, buttocks, and lower back; massages the internal organs; stimulates the nervous system; adjusts the alignment of the pelvis; develops subtle awareness of the interrelationships among the legs, pelvis, abdomen, and lower back.

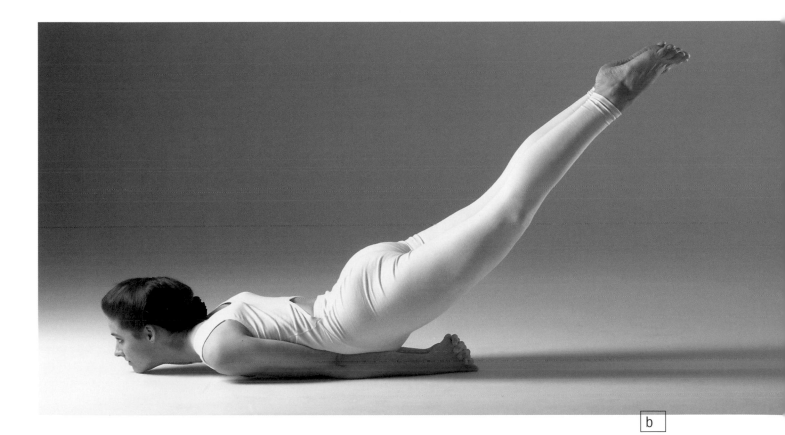

b

Boat Pose (Navasana or Naukasana)

a) Lying on your abdomen, extend the arms overhead alongside the ears. Stretch out through the legs, keeping the feet hip-width apart.

b) Inhaling and lengthening from the navel center, lift the legs, upper body, and arms. Keep the arms alongside the ears. Breathe in the pose as you stretch up and away from the center of the body. Imagine that the arms and legs are infinitely long and that you are floating effortlessly on the breath. With each inhalation stretch further and project the energy of the navel out through the fingers and toes; with each exhalation allow yourself to open more, releasing tension in the shoulders and pelvis. Before releasing the pose, inhale and stretch a little further. Then exhale down and relax.

▶Benefits: Invigorating; strengthens the back muscles; improves circulation to the abdominal organs.

Boat Pose

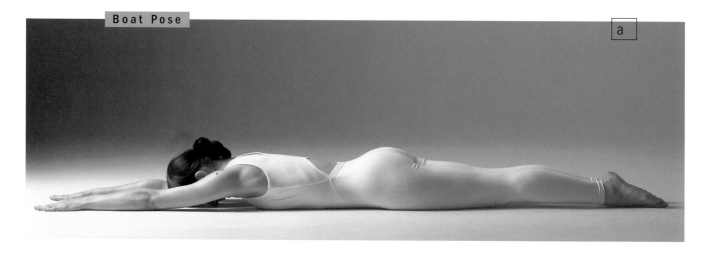

a

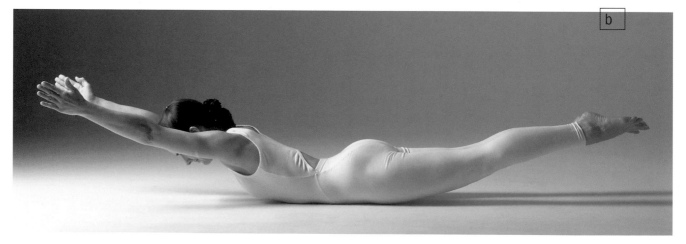

b

15

Knees-to-Chest Pose (Pavanamuktasana)

To counter the intense stretch of the preceding backward bends, lie on your back and bend the knees toward the chest. With your hands, gently draw the thighs toward the abdomen and press the tailbone toward the floor. Then rock gently from side to side, releasing tension and massaging the lower back.

▶ Benefits: Releases tension in the lower back and the hips.

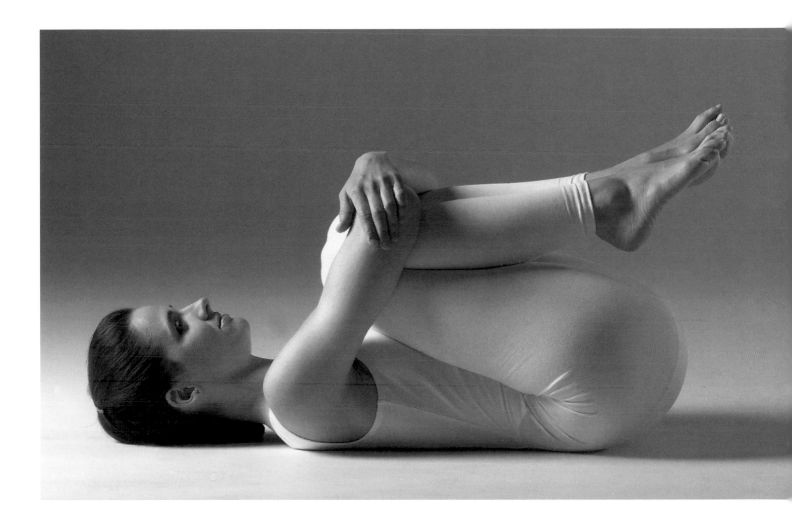

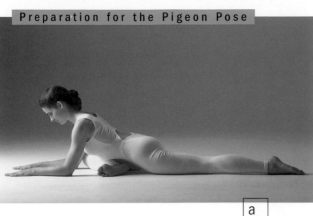

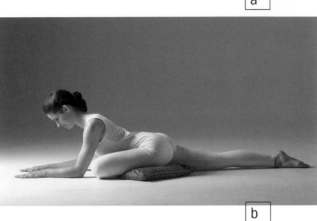

a

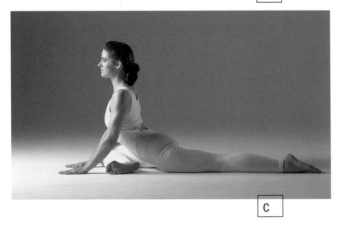

b

c

►<u>Benefits</u>: Improves flexibility and pelvic alignment by stretching the hip rotators and hip flexors; excellent preparation for meditation postures and backward bends.

16

Preparation for the Pigeon Pose
(Kapotasana)

a) Begin on your hands and knees. Bring the right knee forward between the hands and shift the right foot under you to the left. The heel of the right foot is beneath the left side of the pelvis or abdomen. Next, extend the left leg directly behind you and release the pelvis toward the floor.

Slide the hands forward and lower the elbows to the floor. Keep the back of the pelvis level and lower it equally on each side (the groin or abdomen may press against the heel on the left). Release further by lengthening the rear leg, straightening the arms, and lowering the head to the floor.

b) Avoid strain in the knee by adjusting the leg position. If you find the stretch too intense to enjoy, place a cushion or a folded blanket under the thigh and groin of the straight leg and/or the buttock of the bent leg. The support will help you relax. Let the breath be full and deep as you center and relax in the pose.

c) To intensify the stretch, slowly straighten the arms and walk the hands back toward the knee. Lengthen the spine, press the chest forward, and arch up. Elongate the neck and look directly forward. Breathe in the pose as you relax resistance and become steady and comfortable.

To release, sit off to the side and bring the legs together. Move and stretch the legs; then come back to your hands and knees and repeat on the other side.

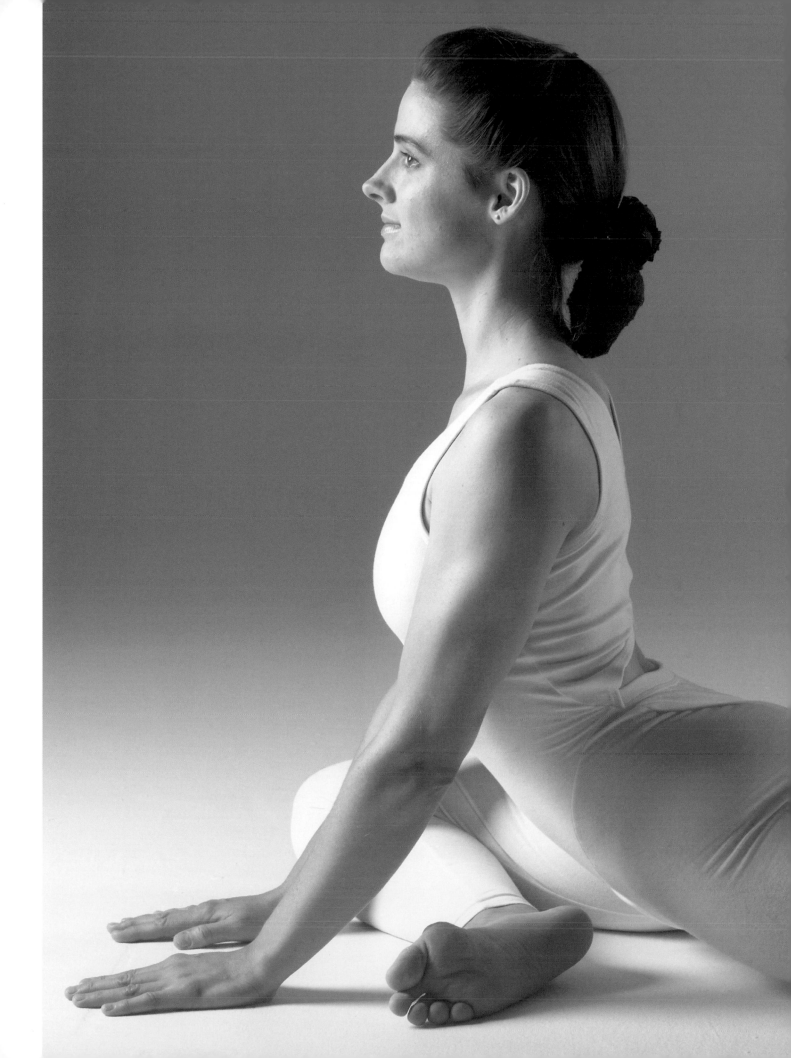

SEATED POSTURES AND
FORWARD BENDS

The seated postures and forward bends strongly work the legs, pelvis, and back. In all of these poses strive to lengthen and elongate the spine, stretching down through the tailbone and up through the top of the head. In the forward bends, rotate the pelvis and stretch forward from the hips, not the waist. Breathe evenly and deeply in all these poses. These postures are calming to the nervous system and soothing to the mind.

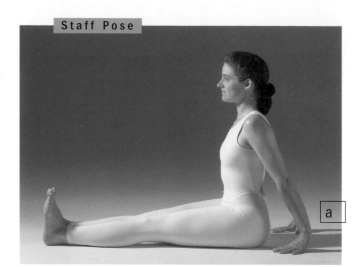

Staff Pose

a

Staff Pose (Dandasana)

a) Sit with the legs together and straight out in front of you. Place the fingertips on the floor slightly behind the hips, with the fingers pointed forward. Inhaling, press down through the fingers, and at the same time lift the lower back, lengthening through the crown of the head. Continue to breathe as you press the back of the legs into the floor, flex the ankles, and extend out through the heels. Lift the chest and ribs while bringing the shoulders back and down. Look straight forward and breathe evenly as you center yourself in the pose. Hold for 5–10 breaths.

b) In this as in other sitting postures, if your lower back collapses, sit on firm cushions or folded blankets to help maintain the natural curve of the lower back and straighten the spine.

c) If your hands reach the floor comfortably, place the palms on the floor alongside the hips.

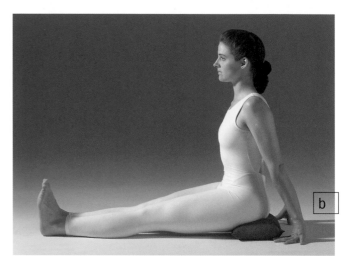

b

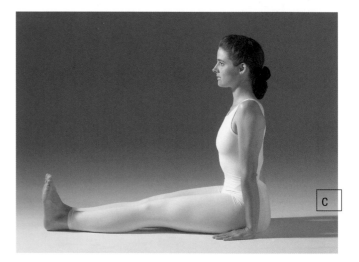

c

▶<u>Benefits</u>: Improves alignment, lower back strength, and awareness of the position of the pelvis and spine. The staff pose is the foundation for other seated postures.

18

Head-to-Knee Pose (Janu Shirshasana)

a) Sit on the floor in the staff pose. (Use a cushion, if necessary, to avoid rounding the lower back.) Bend the left knee and place the sole of the foot against the inner right thigh. Face the right leg, lengthening the torso and keeping the spine erect. Inhale and lift the chest, then exhale and bend from the right hip out over the extended leg, sliding the hands gradually along the floor on either side. Now place the hands on the leg and inhale as you elongate the spine, lift and flatten the lower back, and press the back of the leg toward the floor. Let the neck be long and relaxed.

b) To deepen the stretch, continue to bend forward from the hip and lower the torso toward the leg. Let the hands slide further forward and hold the ankle or toes, or wrap the hands around the foot. If the hands don't easily reach the foot, catch the foot with a strap. Finally, widen and lengthen the back and release the upper body toward the leg. If flexibility allows, stretch the face onto the shin. Breathe and center yourself in the pose. To come out, inhale, flatten the back, and stretch out and up as you slide the hands back toward the pelvis. Repeat on the other side.

▶ Benefits: Stretches the hamstrings and back; improves hip flexibility and pelvic alignment; tones the abdomen; quiets and soothes the mind.

Head-to-Knee Pose

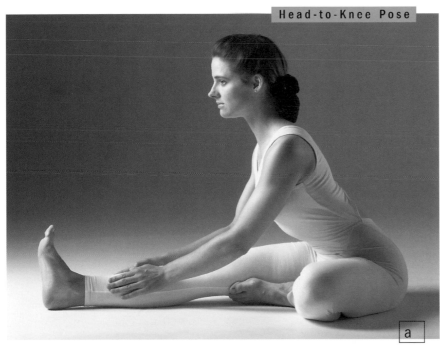

a

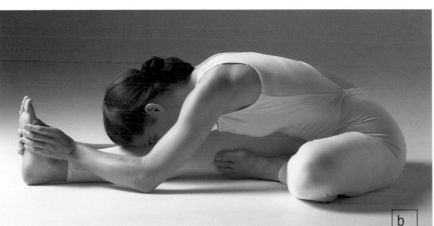

b

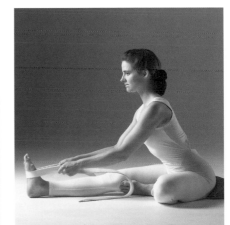

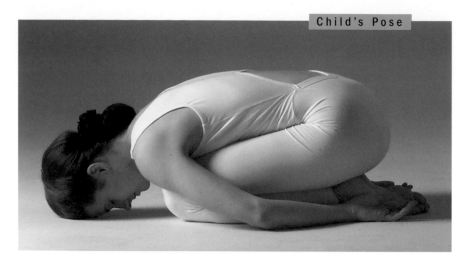

19

Child's Pose (Balasana)

Following the seated bend you may want to again rest in the child's pose. Sit in a kneeling position with the tops of the feet on the floor and the buttocks resting on the heels. With an erect spine, exhale and bend forward from the hips, folding the abdomen to the thighs. Lower the forehead to the floor and rest the arms alongside the body, palms turned up. Feel the motion of the breath against the thighs and at the sides of the rib cage. Relax until the breath is steady and smooth and the mind is ready to continue. If the posture is uncomfortable you may need to spread the knees slightly, or place cushions under the ankles or the back of the thighs. An alternative is to lie on the back, bringing the knees to the chest. To come out of this pose and into the next one, lift the head, flatten the back, and return to an upright posture.

▶Benefits: Relieves lower back tension; gently stretches the spine; massages the abdominal organs; refreshes the legs; quiets the mind.

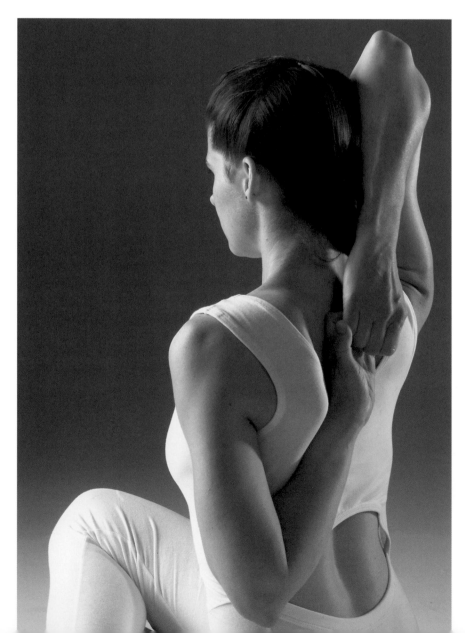

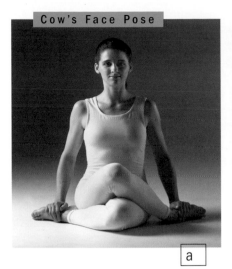

Cow's Face Pose

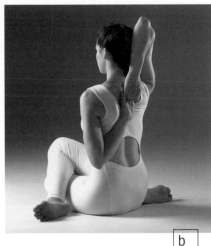

a

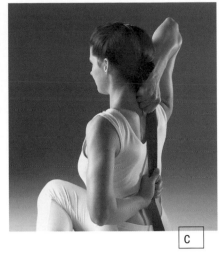

b

c

20

Cow's Face Pose
(Gomukhasana)

a) Sit in the staff pose. Fold the left
leg under the right, placing the left
heel on the floor near the right hip.
Wrap the right leg over the left so
that the right foot is near the outside
of the left hip. Adjust the legs so
that the right knee is directly above
the left. Rest on both sitting bones
and sit up straight, lifting through
the top of the head. Place the hands
on the feet.

▶ Benefits: Improves flexibility in
the shoulders and hips; supports
an erect, steady posture; facilitates
diaphragmatic breathing.

b) Bring the right arm overhead.
Bend the elbow, and reach back and
down along the spine with the
hand. Next, bring the left forearm to
the lower back, stretching the hand
as far as possible to the right side
before sliding it up the back to clasp
the right hand.

c) If the hands don't reach one
another, hold a belt or strap
between them to act as an extension
of the arms. Lift the spine, and relax
and open from the center of the
chest. Draw the left shoulder back
and lengthen through the right
elbow. Without straining either
shoulder joint, move the elbows
toward the axis of the spine and
bring the hands closer together.
Breathe freely for several breaths,
then release the arms slowly and
unwind the legs. Repeat on the
other side.

Butterfly Pose

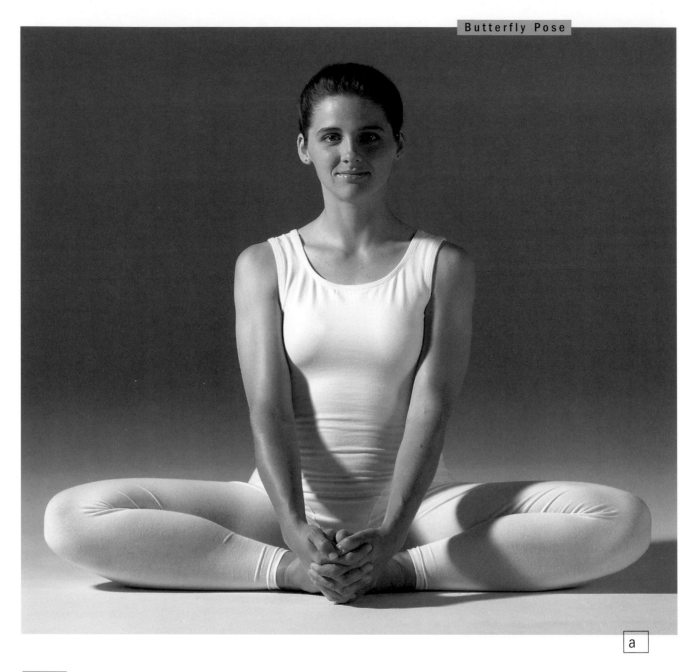

a

Butterfly Pose (Baddha Konasana)

a) Sit erect with the soles of the feet together and the heels close to the pelvis (use a cushion, if necessary, to avoid rounding the lower back). Clasp the hands around the feet, pressing the knees down. Lift the lower back and extend upward through the whole spine. The sitting bones press into the floor. Lift the breastbone, extending through the neck and crown of the head. Now watch the breath as you release resistance and become steady and comfortable in the pose.

b) To increase the stretch, lift the lower back and tilt the pelvis forward. Exhale and bend forward from the hips, drawing the pubic bones down and back between the thighs. Press the inner thighs down toward the floor.

c) In the final stage of the pose the torso is lowered onto the feet and the head rests on the floor. But wherever you are in the bend, watch the breath as you release resistance, and deepen into the pose.

▶ <u>Benefits</u>: Tones the pelvic floor; increases flexibility of hips, pelvis, inner thighs, lower back, knees, and ankles; normalizes reproductive system and urinary system. This pose is particularly helpful for menstrual problems.

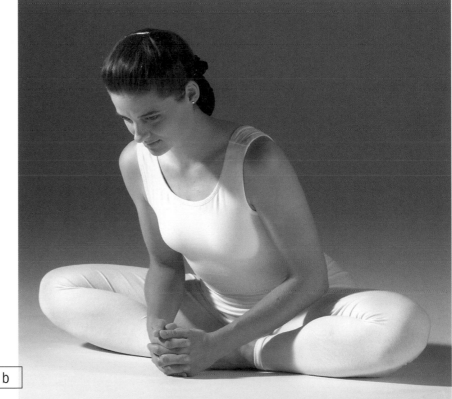

b

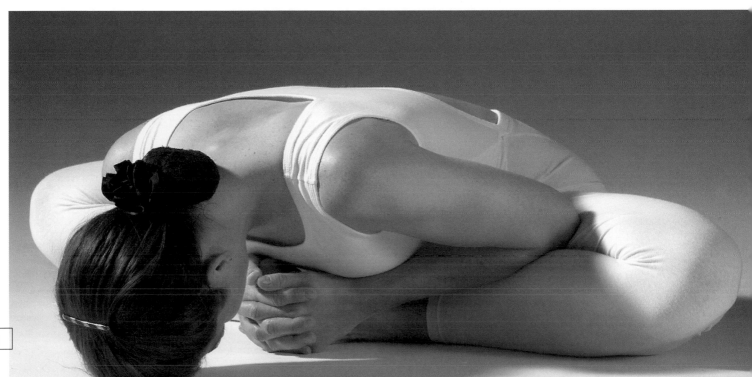

c

Hip-Balancing Sequence

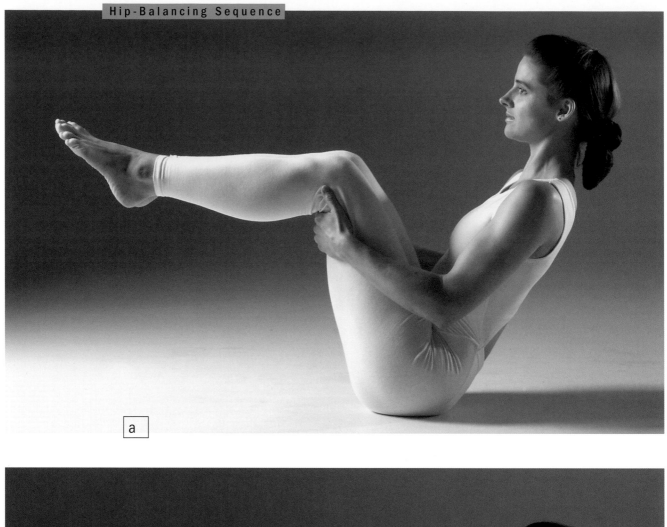

a

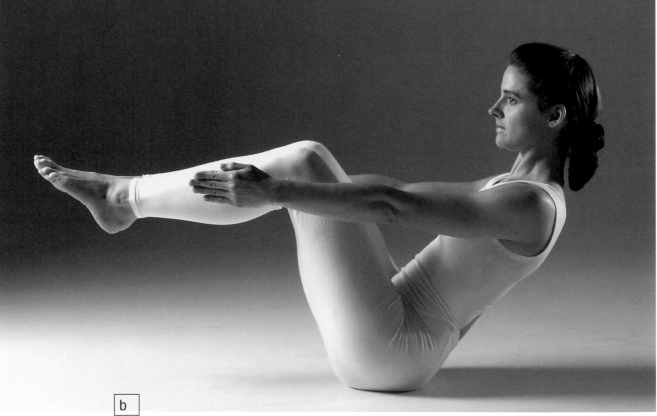

b

22

Hip-Balancing Sequence

a) From the staff pose, bend both knees and draw them toward the chest, keeping the knees together. Hold behind the knees, lean back slightly, and lift the lower legs parallel to the floor. Lift the lower back and chest, lengthen through the spine, and extend through the top of the head. Keep the knees and ankles together and the shoulders down. Hold for about 5 breaths.

b) To deepen the pose, let go of the knees and straighten the arms alongside the legs. Keep the knees and ankles together, the lower legs parallel to the floor, and the torso erect and pulled toward the thighs. Hold for about 5 breaths.

c) Finally, to further strengthen the abdomen, straighten the knees and angle the legs toward the ceiling. Lengthen the spine, lift the chest, and lower the shoulders. Hold for about 5 breaths.

▶Benefits: Strengthens the abdomen and lumbar spine; helps with spinal alignment; improves meditation postures.

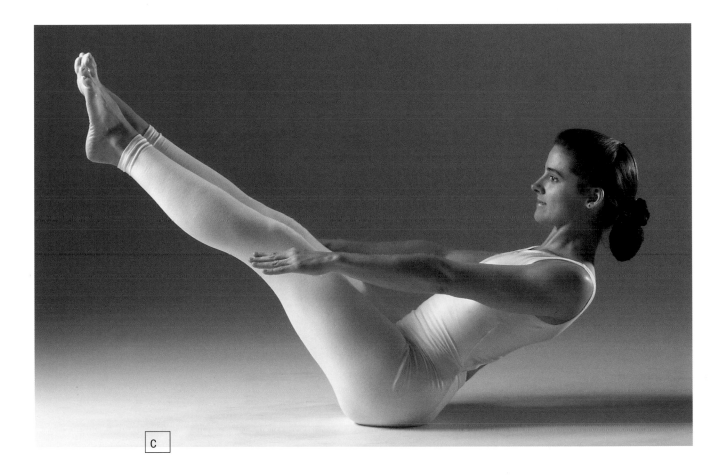

C

23

Seated Spinal Twist
(Ardha Matsyendrasana)

a) Sit in the staff pose. Fold the right leg under the left, placing the right heel on the floor near the left hip. Raise the left knee and step your foot across the right leg, placing the left foot flat on the floor near the outside of the right knee or thigh. Straighten the spine. Place the hands on the floor behind you, opening the shoulders. Use the hands to press into the floor, elongating the spine.

b) Wrap the right arm around the left knee and hold the knee in the crook of the elbow. Shift the abdomen across the thigh. Then exhale and twist to the left. Begin the twist from deep in the abdomen and move up through the rib cage, shoulders, neck, and head. As you hold the twist, lift the lower back and lengthen through the spine with each inhalation. Deepen the twist with each exhalation.

c) To further deepen the twist bring the right elbow to the outside of the left knee. Use the pressure of the arm against the leg to accentuate the twist. The right hand may be at the chest, or you may open the elbow and reach back to grasp the left foot or ankle. In either position keep the spine elongated, the shoulders down, and both sitting bones grounded. Inhale deeply into the abdomen despite the resistance you may feel from the twist. When you are ready to come out, release the head, then the shoulders, chest, pelvis, and legs. Repeat the pose on the other side.

▶ Benefits: Strengthens the diaphragm; improves circulation to the abdominal organs; stimulates and balances digestive, reproductive, and eliminative systems; increases flexibility of hips, shoulders, and spine; improves all sitting postures.

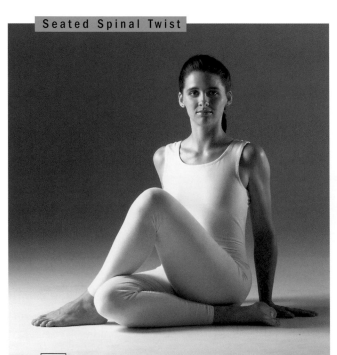

Seated Spinal Twist

a

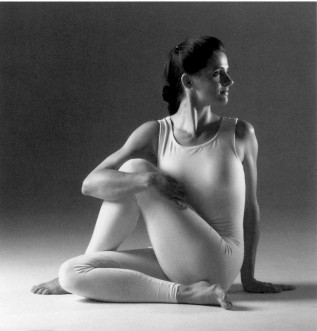

b

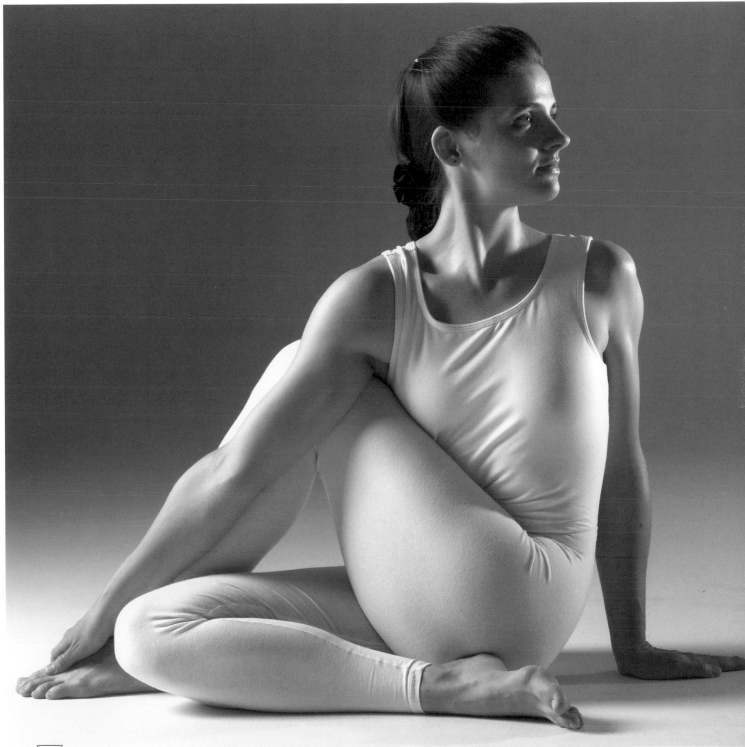

C

INVERSIONS AND
BACK-RELIEVERS

This section includes two inverted postures and three poses intended to relieve any remaining muscle strain (especially in the lower back) prior to relaxation. Inverted postures are a unique and important part of yoga practice. With legs raised and head lowered, the effects of gravity on the circulatory system are reversed and a rich supply of arterial blood is brought to the brain, the cranial nerves, and the glands of the upper body. Inversions also drain venous blood pooled in the legs and abdomen, bringing it back to the heart. With regular practice breathing is deepened and internal organs are massaged. Psychologically, inverted poses are relaxing and they build confidence. If we can remain centered while our world is turned upside down, we will develop internal strength and poise.

Caution: Inverted poses are important, but they need to be learned systematically in order to prevent injury. Follow the instructions carefully, and if you feel strain in the head, neck, eyes, or ears, come out of the pose.

Before ending the sequence it is wise to do a few stretches that help unwind the body. This will provide an opportunity to rest, revitalize, and reap the rewards of your practice. Use these stretches to release any remaining stress so that you'll feel completely comfortable and balanced as you begin the final relaxation in the corpse pose. Working with this in mind, avoid undue effort. Allow the body, nervous system, and mind to become calm, quiet, and balanced.

Rocking Chair

Sit on a carpeted surface or mat with the knees raised and feet flat. Make sure there is space behind as well as in front of you. Clasp each thigh just behind the knee and round the entire spine (including the lower back) like a rocker on a rocking chair. Keeping the spine rounded, gently roll backward toward the shoulders, as you raise and straighten the legs. Then roll forward to the starting position, adding momentum by bending the knees. Be sure to keep the lower back rounded as you come forward to make it easier to return to the upright position. Repeat 10 or more times.

▶Benefits: Massages the back and spinal column, improves coordination and balance; prepares the body for inverted postures.

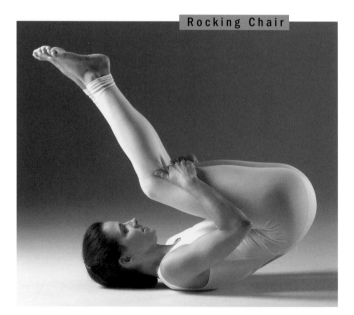

Rocking Chair

25

Inverted Action Pose (Viparita Karani)

a) To prepare for inverted postures, and to gain some of their benefits with only a modest effort, lie on the floor with the legs raised against a wall. Come into the pose by sitting on the floor with the outside of one hip and shoulder against the wall and your hands behind you on the floor. Lean back, bend the knees toward the chest, and rotate the body so that the tailbone is near the wall and the top of the head is pointed away from it. Extend the legs vertically against the wall and rest the back and the head on the floor. The arms may be alongside the body or you may rest the arms above the head, opening the elbows. Hold and breathe, remaining in the pose for 1–3 minutes. Release by bending the knees and rolling to the side.

Inverted Action Pose

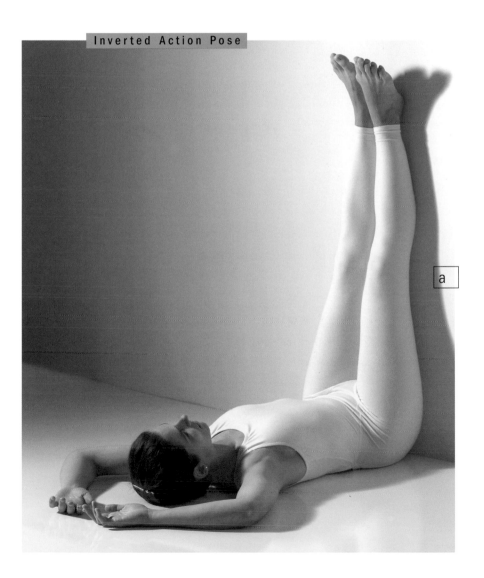

a

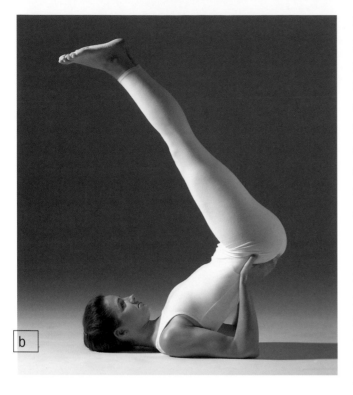

b

b) When you are ready to practice the inverted action pose, start from the beginning position of the previous pose, the rocking chair. Roll backward, straightening the knees and bringing the legs overhead; then slide your elbows underneath and support the lower back with your hands. The upper arms rest on the floor. Carefully shift your weight from side to side, drawing the upper arms and shoulder blades toward one another under the body. The torso extends away from the head at about 45 degrees.

c) Shift the weight of the pelvis further onto the hands. Note that the chest is never raised vertically in this posture. When the pelvis is securely resting on the forearms, then raise the legs until they are vertical to the floor. The heels of the hands are against the iliac crest (the bony ridge at the back of the pelvis). Though the weight is felt at the elbows, it is distributed through the whole surface of the upper arm, from elbow to shoulder. Adjust the hands, reposition the elbows, open the chest, and relax the neck to make the posture comfortable. Deepen your breathing as you hold the pose. Then watch the breath and center your attention. Changes in circulation patterns will produce a mild pressure in the head that should pass quickly, followed by a sense of pleasant fullness. If the pressure is aggravating, come out of the pose and consult with a qualified teacher or health practitioner. Start by holding for 10–20 seconds. Gradually increase the time to one minute or longer.

When you are ready to come out of the pose bring the legs over the head. Bend the knees and support the back with the hands as you round and lower the back one vertebra at a time, finally releasing the legs to the floor. The legs can also be kept straight and lowered to the floor. In that case, grip the floor with the lower back as the legs descend; if the back comes away from the floor, bend the legs.

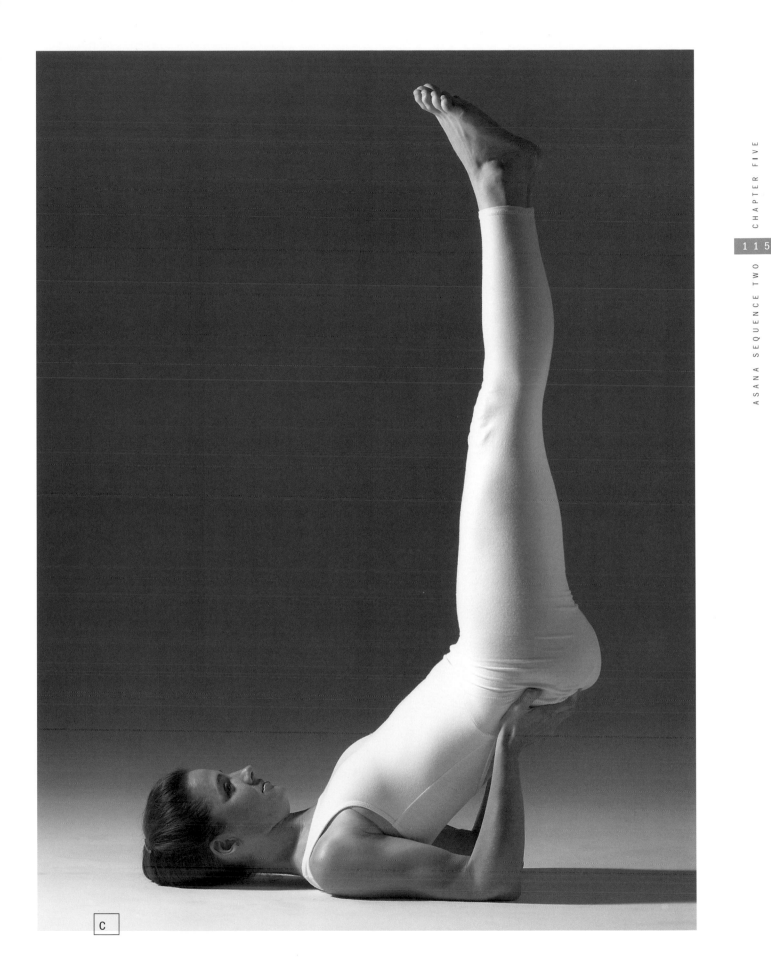

C

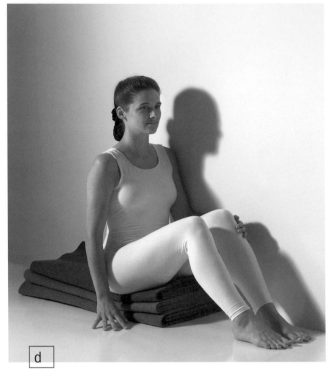

d

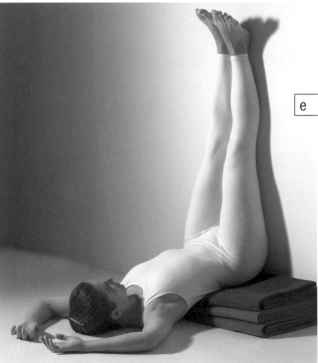

e

d) The inverted action pose can also be practiced against a wall, using blankets or cushions to elevate the pelvis and lower back. This variation makes the pose more accessible for those who cannot support the pelvis with the arms. Begin by sitting sideways on cushions or a stack of folded blankets. Experiment to find the right cushion height and placement.

e) Turn your body and raise the legs onto the wall, adjusting the blankets underneath the hips and lower back so that they provide comfortable support. The hips are square and both buttocks touch the wall. Lengthen the spine, rest the backs of the shoulders on the floor, and open the chest. The arms rest above the head with elbows open to the side. Relax and breathe. Start by holding the pose for 30 seconds, and gradually increase to 1–3 minutes.

Caution: Do not practice either version of the inverted action pose if you are menstruating, if you are pregnant, or if you have high blood pressure or heart problems. Other contraindications include a detached retina, certain ear problems, recent abdominal surgery, or an injury to the spine (seek advice).

▶Benefits: The downward flow of blood cleanses the lower limbs and nourishes the upper body, neck, and head; improves concentration; removes fatigue; relieves varicose veins; strengthens the diaphragm. A most beneficial pose for daily practice.

Reclining Twist Variation

Lie on the back, arms on the floor directly out from the shoulders, palms down. Keeping the right leg straight, bend the left knee and place the foot on the floor near the pelvis. Lift the pelvis and slide the right hip further underneath to realign the torso and permit a deeper twist. Now raise the left knee and twist the pelvis to the right, bringing the knee toward the floor. Turn the head to the left, and press the left shoulder toward the floor to deepen the twist. Breathe deeply in the stretch. Begin by holding for 15–20 seconds, then repeat on the opposite side.

▶Benefits: Increases flexibility in the entire spine; improves digestion, and tones the organs of the abdomen. This and the two following stretches will relieve back discomfort and help close this sequence of asanas.

Reclining Twist Variation

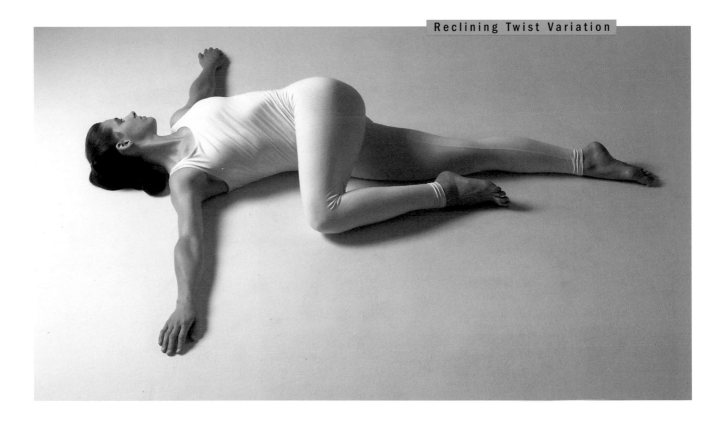

Knees-to-Chest Pose (Pavanamuktasana)

Lie on the back with the legs together. Raising the right knee, wrap both hands around the leg and pull the knee toward the chest. Keep the lower back firm and do not lift the left leg, pelvis, or upper back and shoulders from the floor. Hold for 10–15 seconds and repeat on the opposite side. Then raise both knees and clasp the hands around both legs, pulling the knees toward the chest. Soften the lower back and abdomen. Breathe evenly into the lower abdomen and hold for 10–15 seconds.

▶Benefits: Releases lower back tension and massages the abdomen.

Arch Pose

Lie on the back, knees raised and feet hip-width apart. The arms rest toward the feet, palms down. Exhale and press the abdomen and the lower back into the floor, tilting the pelvis until the lower vertebrae of the lumbar spine begin to lift. Roll up and down the spine, one vertebra at a time, starting with just the lower part of the spine and gradually moving higher. Release slowly, lengthening the lower back and relaxing the buttocks. Repeat 5–7 times or until back tension has resolved.

▶Benefits: Increases flexibility of the spine; releases lower back tension; develops more subtle control of the muscles of the lower back, abdomen, thighs, and pelvis.

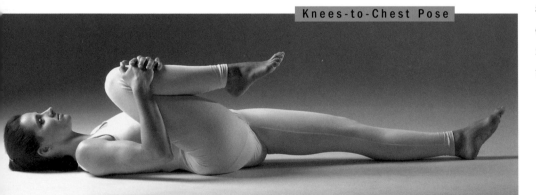

Knees-to-Chest Pose

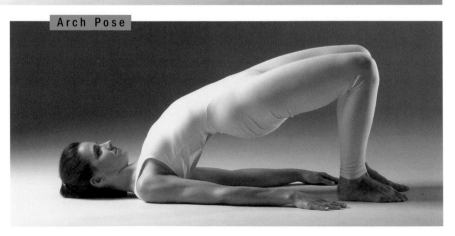

Arch Pose

Corpse Pose (Shavasana)

Lie on your back on a firm, flat surface. Rest the legs about 12 14 inches apart. Rest the arms 6–8 inches from the sides, palms turned upward (they may, however, roll inward). Bring the shoulder blades slightly together, opening the chest and relaxing the arms. Use a thin cushion to support the neck and head. If there is discomfort in the lower back, support the knees with a folded blanket. Close your eyes and let the body become completely still. Use a relaxation exercise from chapter 8, or simply focus on the flow of the breath. Relax for about 10 minutes but do not drift into sleep.

When you have finished relaxing, stretch the arms overhead on the floor, bring the feet together, and inhale, reaching down through the feet and out through the hands and fingers in a symmetrical stretch. When you're ready, fold the knees to the chest and roll onto your left side. Rest for a moment on your side, then sit up.

▶ Benefits: Deeply relaxing. Calms the mind; rejuvenates and refreshes the body and mind; balances the nervous system. Follows all yoga sequences.

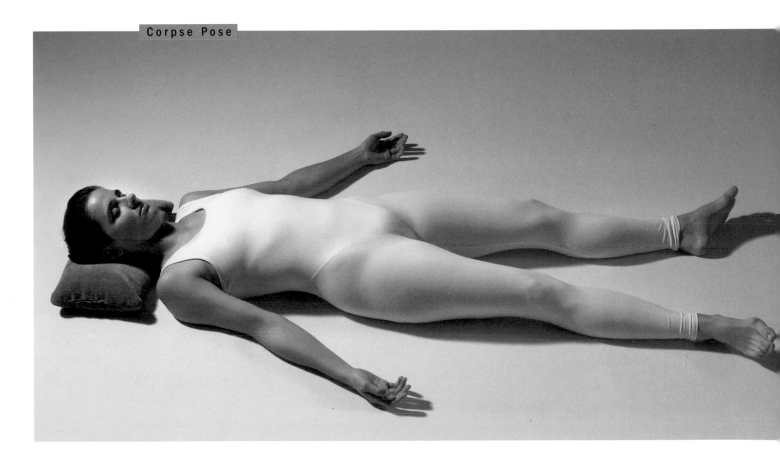

Corpse Pose

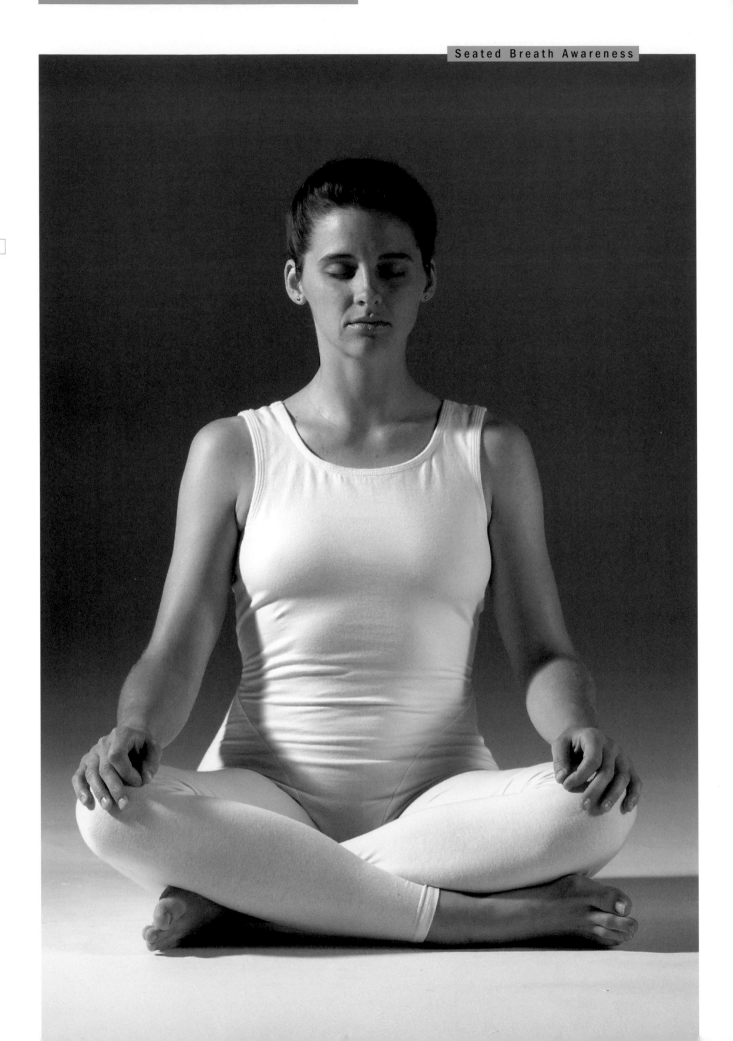

30

Seated Breath Awareness

Sit in any comfortable cross-legged position (use cushions to help). Close your eyes and turn your attention to your breath. Observe the flow of the breath for a few minutes, establishing smooth diaphragmatic breathing. Then relax the body and sit quietly with your awareness centered in the flow of the breath. When you have learned the meditation methods in chapter 9, then incorporate them here. Finally, when you're ready to turn your attention outward, acknowledge the presence of stillness and awareness within you, and gently open your eyes.

Moving On

Asana Sequence Two is both comprehensive and systematic, and you will find yourself returning to it. But you may also find yourself wanting to vary your routine and tailor your practice session to your individual needs. For example, you may want to concentrate on a particular problem such as weak shoulders, or perhaps you'd like to spend more time on a particular aspect of practice such as forward bends. Or if you have very little time this week—how should you modify your practice to fit into 20 minutes? Chapter 6 provides suggestions for working with problem areas and an outline for designing your own practice.

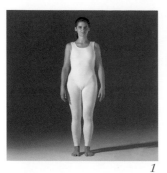

1

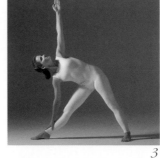

2

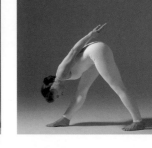

3

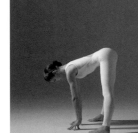

4

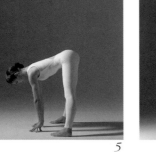

5

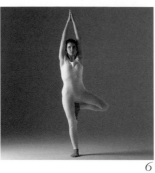

6

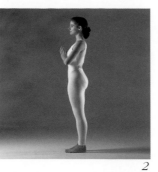

7

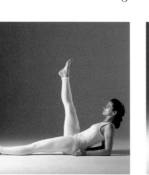

8

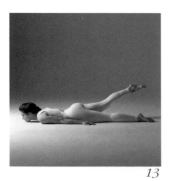

9

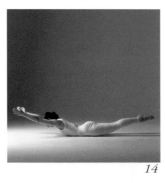

10

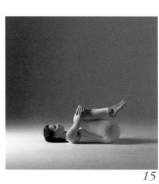

11

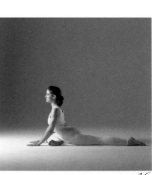

12

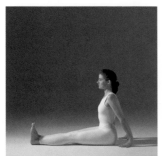

13

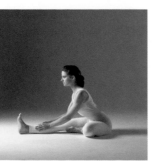

14

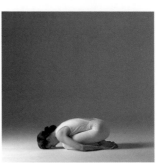

15

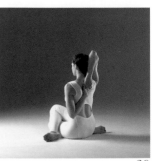

16

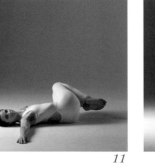

17

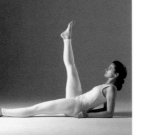

18

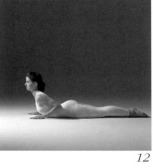

19

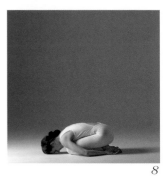

20

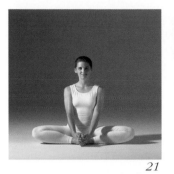

21

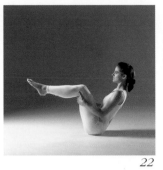

22

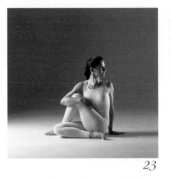

23

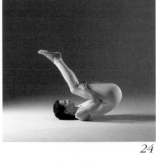

24

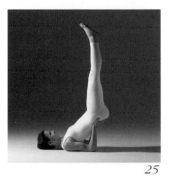

25

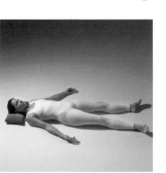

26

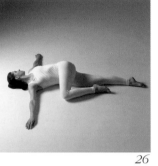

27

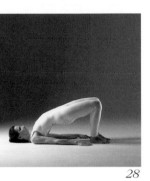

28

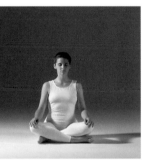

29

30

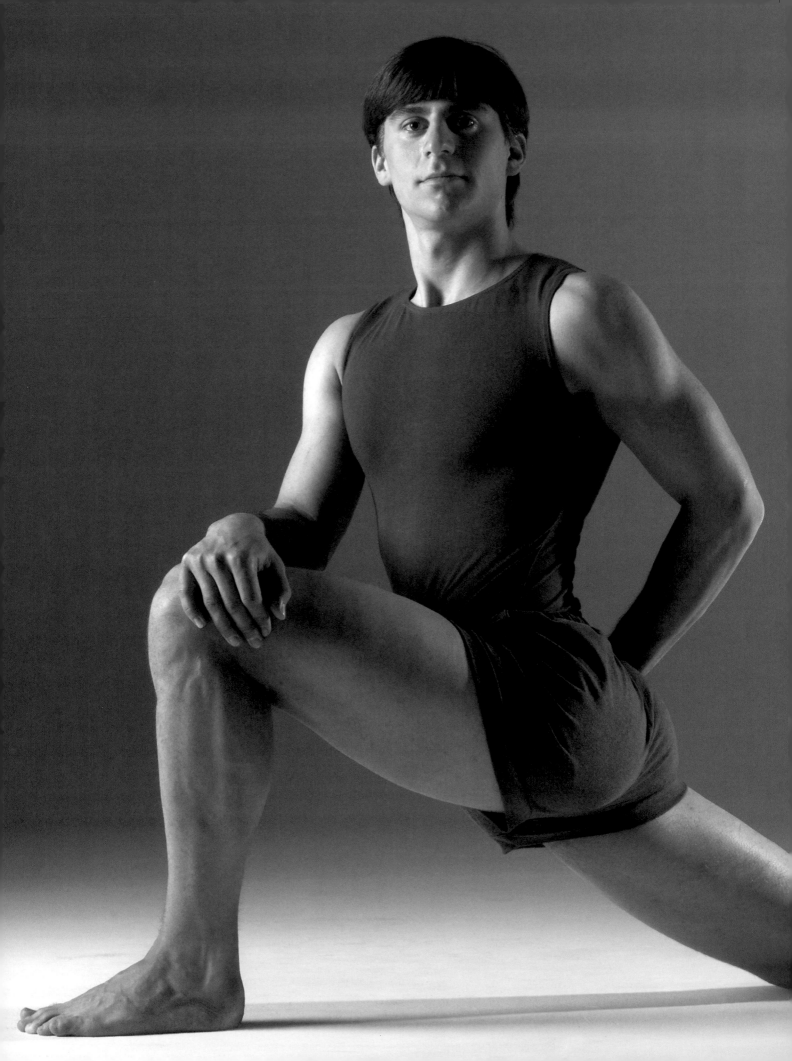

CHAPTER SIX

PROGRESS IN PRACTICE

Do not kill the instinct of the body
for the glory of the pose.

——— *Vanda Scaravelli*

IF we cultivate our yoga practice it will bring us closer and closer to a balance point, to a state of stability, ease, and inner stillness from which health and happiness blossom. But unless our practice continues to unfold it eventually begins to calcify.

Perhaps you are ready to deepen your practice with pranayama, meditation, and changes in lifestyle, all of which are the subject of chapters to come; or perhaps you're also ready to advance in the postures. In this chapter you'll find guidelines for customizing your asana practice, additional work for common problem areas, and hints for deepening your experience in all postures.

DEVELOPING YOUR OWN HATHA PRACTICE

After you have learned the Asana Sequences One and Two and are comfortable with them, you may find yourself wanting to do more. For example, you may notice recalcitrant tension in the shoulders and neck, or you may see how tight hamstrings hamper all forward bends, and decide to focus on postures that target these areas. The routines we have learned so far may work just fine—but your own tailor-made sequence will keep you inspired and at the same time deepen your experience of the postures.

To customize your practice, first ask yourself, "What are my intentions and goals? What are the obstacles I face?" Goals are both long-term and short-term. For example, a long-term goal might be to improve your health, and a short-term goal might be to strengthen the abdomen—in which case you would include leglifts and boat poses in your routine. Or you may have the general goal of enhancing your meditation practice, and the short-term goal of improving hip flexibility—so you spend more time with hip-opening postures. Consider also the time that is available to you. If your inclination and interest is pranayama practice, choose asanas to facilitate breathing and sitting, but spend more time with systematic breath training. If your interest is meditation, let your preparation focus on those asanas, breathing, and relaxation techniques that deepen and support that goal. And be aware that goals can evolve over time as your capacity and understanding grow, so be flexible in your thinking as well as your body—and change your practice as needed.

The next step is to evaluate the time available to you as well as your inclinations and tendencies. If you are the type that suddenly realizes it's breakfast time and you've barely gotten started, it may be helpful to establish a sequence of poses (write them down!) that can easily be done in an hour, and then stick to it. On the other hand, if your pattern is to rush through everything, lightly brushing the surface, you might focus on a few deep calming stretches, lengthening your stay in each. This approach to customizing your practice requires honest self-evaluation.

Whatever your goals and situation, design your practice with the following general sequence of postures in mind:

- ► Centering and Warming Up
- ► Standing Poses
- ► Abdominal Strengthening and Energizing
- ► Seated, Prone, and Supine Poses
- ► Backward Bends
- ► Forward Bends
- ► Twists
- ► Inverted Poses
- ► Relaxation

Within this framework you can construct a tailor-made sequence that addresses your individual needs. It can be long or short, it can focus on abdominal strengthening with only a few poses from the other categories, or it can address the hip-opening aspects of forward bends and spend minimal time on other poses—the possibilities are many. But regardless of your focus, every set of postures should strive for balance. We need to work in all the major areas and in all directions. And remember that many postures require preparation and/or counter-poses. A backward bend like the locust pose or cobra pose, for example, begs for a gentle forward-bend counterpose like the child's pose, so be sure to include postures from all the major categories regardless of your focus.

Put yourself in the role of a teacher. If you develop a sequence (or at least an outline), you'll find it easier to practice on those days when you don't quite have the energy to decide what to do next. Working from a plan takes less discipline than simply winging it. You can create your own sequence or you can modify one of the sequences we've already learned.

The following sections focus on additional work for areas that are particularly problematic: hips, hamstrings, lower back, abdomen, and shoulders. Each begins with a brief overview followed by a list of relevant poses that you have already learned from Asana Sequences One and Two. Use the list to develop a focused practice routine to stretch or strengthen a particular region, and then add the new poses that follow to deepen your work.

ADDITIONAL WORK FOR PROBLEM AREAS

HIPS AND PELVIS

The pelvis, lower spine, and hip joints bear the weight of the upper half of the body, stabilize the relationship between the torso and the legs, and form the framework needed for walking, running, twisting, and bending in all directions. The primary connection between the pelvis and the lower spine takes place at the sacroiliac joints, which lie on either side of the sacrum and are relatively immobile. Their semi-rigid construction firmly anchors the base of the spine, and for the most part the lower spine and pelvis function as a unit.

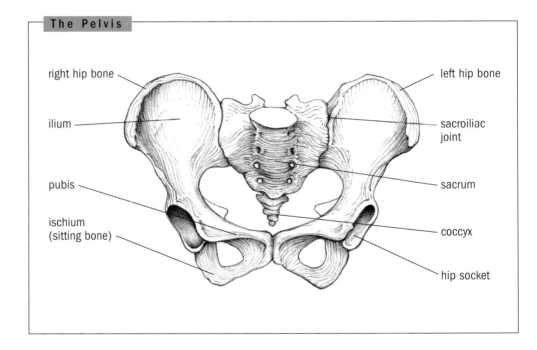

The Pelvis

right hip bone

ilium

pubis

ischium (sitting bone)

left hip bone

sacroiliac joint

sacrum

coccyx

hip socket

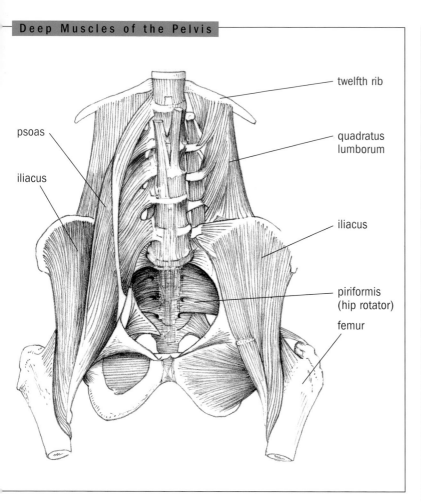

psoas

iliacus

twelfth rib

quadratus
lumborum

iliacus

piriformis
(hip rotator)

femur

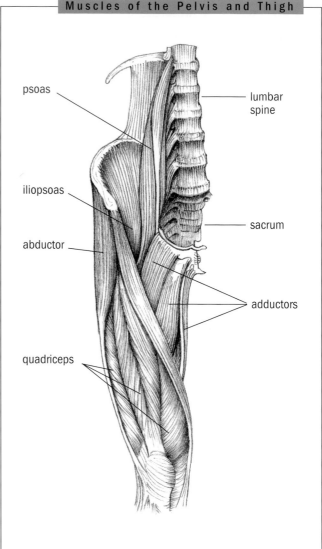

psoas

iliopsoas

abductor

quadriceps

lumbar
spine

sacrum

adductors

The thighs, on the other hand, are joined to the pelvis in ball-and-socket joints that are among the most mobile joints of the body. This allows for a wide range of movements at the hip—the thigh can move forward and backward and side to side, and it can be rotated so that it turns in and out. As might be expected in an area that includes such different functions, many muscle groups contribute to flexibility and strength. The hamstrings in the back of the thighs, the quadriceps in front, the adductors of the inner thighs, the abductors behind and to the sides, the rotators, and the hip flexors (iliopsoas muscles), which are located deep in the pelvis, all move the thighs in relation to the pelvis. Finally, the abdominal muscles support the front of the body and help with proper alignment of the pelvis and lower spine.

Unless the hip joints are exercised regularly in all directions, problems such as stiffness, pain, or chronic foreshortening of their muscles will invariably appear. Many of the following exercises are stretches designed to open up this area. When the problem of stiff joints, however, is accompanied by tight hamstrings and a stiff lower back, you will also need to work on these areas as well. Keep in mind that tight muscles are often compensating for weak ones; a well-rounded program that includes strengthening exercises (such as the standing poses along with deep stretches) will restore balance to the musculature and bring a normal range of motion more quickly than specific exercises in isolation. A number of postures in Asana Sequences One and Two address these problems:

 Lunge pose p.35

 Leg cradles p.39

 Seated forward stretch p.41

 Spinal twists pp.42, 44, 92, 110

 Preparation for the pigeon pose p.100

 Cow's face pose p.105

Butterfly pose p.106

Standing poses Chapters 3 & 5

Side Angle Pose

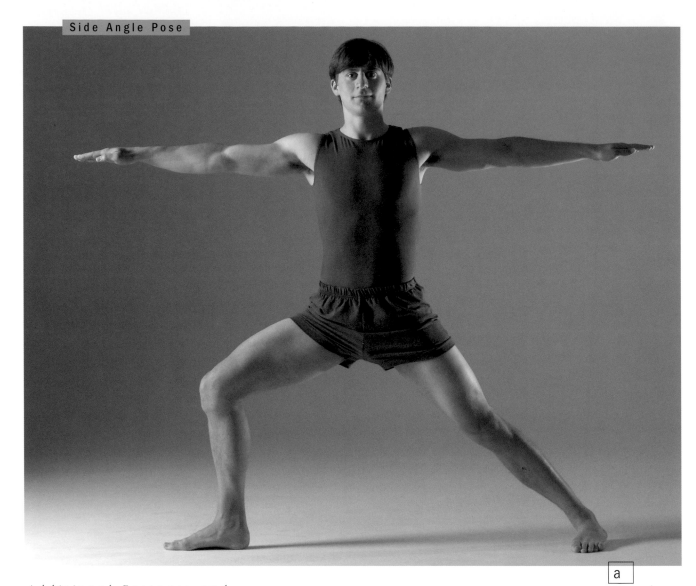

a

Additional Postures and
Stretches for the Hips and Pelvis

Side Angle Pose (Parshvakonasana)

The standing poses are excellent for the hips and pelvis because they develop strength and flexibility, and because they integrate your awareness with postural movements. The side angle pose increases mobility deep in the hip joints; strengthens the quadriceps and other muscles of the legs and pelvis; stretches muscles along the entire side of the body; and expands the chest.

a) Stand with the feet about a leg's-length apart. Turn the right foot out 90 degrees and the left slightly in, hips and chest facing forward. Inhaling, stretch the arms straight out from the shoulders, palms down, keeping the shoulders broad and down away from the ears. Exhaling, bend the right knee until it is directly over the ankle. Steady the pose and relax the breath.

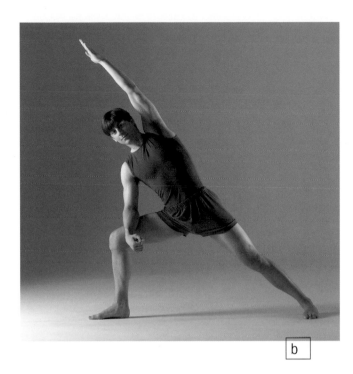

b

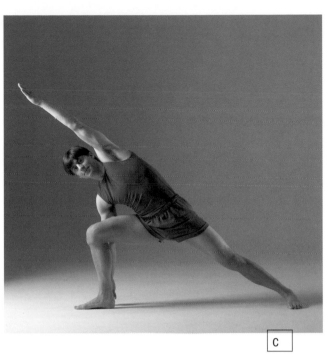

c

b) With the torso still facing forward, exhale, lengthen the spine, and bend to the right, resting the right forearm on the thigh while turning the left palm up and raising the left arm parallel to the side of the head. Then further open the chest and abdomen by slightly tucking the tailbone and drawing the shoulder blades in. Press the feet firmly into the floor, and lengthen from the left heel through the left fingertips. For stability keep the right knee directly over the ankle, and the outer left foot pressing into the floor.

c) To deepen the pose, stretch the inner thighs away from each other. Then release the right arm from the thigh and place the hand on the floor at the outside of the right foot. Lower the left hip until it is in line with the extended leg and arm, lengthening the stretch through the entire left side. Keep the right arm and leg together, rotating the rib cage and abdomen open, and lifting the chest away from the pelvis. Stretch the left arm; open the left shoulder; and keeping the neck long, look straight ahead, or turn the head to look up. Now breathe steadily as you center yourself in the pose, holding for 3–5 breaths or until you feel ready to come out. Then press through the ball of the right foot, lift the torso, and straighten the leg. Exchange the position of the feet, and repeat on the other side.

Lunge Pose Variations (Banarasana)

The lunge and its variations are excellent postures for correcting pelvic alignment and lower back problems. The iliopsoas muscles, instrumental in flexing the hip, connect the lower spine and pelvis to the thigh bones. These muscles are often tight, and either weaker or more flexible on one side than the other, throwing off the alignment of the pelvis, legs, and spine. The lunge variations stretch the psoas muscles as well as the quadriceps. Healthy, pliable psoas muscles are also a prerequisite for successful backward-bending poses.

Lunge Pose Variations

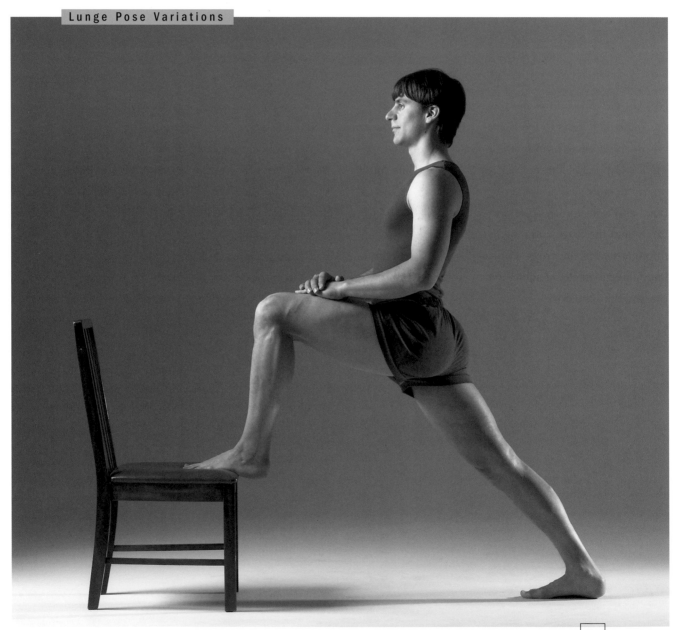

a

a) If the basic lunge pose (p.35) is difficult, try this. Standing about three feet from a chair, place the left foot on the chair seat. Bend the left knee and distribute your weight between the two legs, maintaining an upright spine. Rest the hands on the left thigh. Keep the right leg straight, the heel resting on the foot, and the foot facing forward. Gradually deepen the bend in the hip joint, lowering the pelvis toward the floor. Relax and breathe in the pose; then repeat on the opposite side.

b) The following variation deepens the lunge pose. Begin on your hands and knees, then bring the left foot forward between the hands so that the toes are in line with the fingers. Extend the right leg straight behind you, resting the knee and the top of the foot on the floor. Keep the left knee directly over the ankle with the shin perpendicular to the floor. Lower the pelvis, lengthening the two thighs in opposite directions, and press the chest forward and up. Now bring the toes of the right foot under. Lift the right knee, straighten the leg, and press the heel away from the body. With the knee raised, continue lowering the pelvis toward the floor while pressing the left thigh forward and the right thigh back. Hold and breathe, then repeat on the opposite side.

c) You can also use the weight of the torso to deepen the stretch. Begin in the basic lunge pose with the right knee and top of the foot on the floor. Next, raise the torso perpendicular to the floor and center it over the pelvis. After establishing your balance, slowly lower the pelvis further. Now, maintaining an erect spine, twist to the left. Bring the right hand to the outside of the left knee and wrap the left arm around the back with the hand at the right hip. Hold and breathe deeply into the twist for a number of breaths, then release and repeat on the other side.

d) To deepen the stretch in the quadriceps, start in the basic lunge position with the right leg extended behind. Lift the torso and center yourself over the pelvis. Next, bend the right knee, raising the foot, and reach back with the right hand to grasp it. Hold the foot and establish your balance, keeping the pelvis square to the front. Then exhale and bend forward, lowering the left hand to the floor (or placing it on a support). Draw the right foot toward the buttock, stretching the quadriceps. Center in the pose and breathe smoothly. Then repeat on the opposite side.

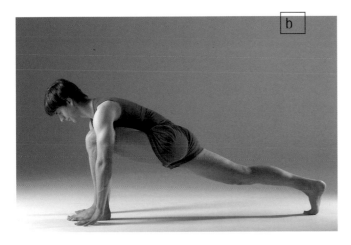

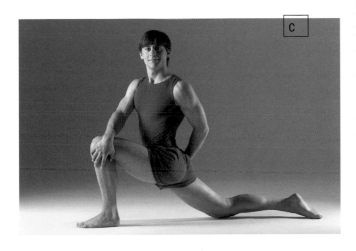

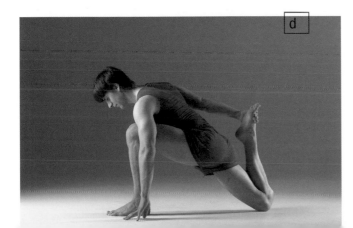

Half Hero Pose Variations

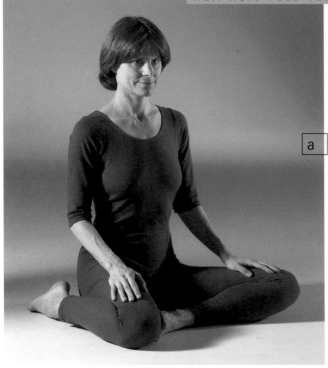

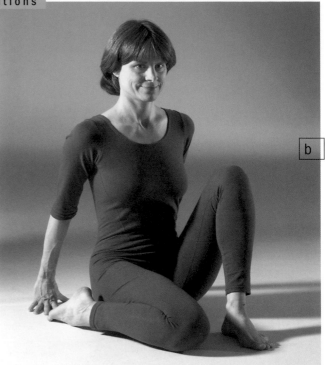

Half Hero Pose Variations (Virasana)

If the quadriceps are tight and the hips, knees, and ankles are stiff, these variations of the hero pose will help. But exercise caution and work slowly with these stretches since they put considerable pressure on the knees and ankles. Throughout all the variations, avoid pain or excessive discomfort in the ankles, knees, or lower back.

a) Sit on the floor with both legs in front of you. Bend the right knee and place the top of the foot alongside the right hip, toes pointing backward (sit on a cushion for support if necessary). Bend the left knee, bringing the sole of the foot to the inner right thigh and releasing the left knee out to the side. Now press the right knee gently into the floor and lengthen the top of the thigh. Hold and breathe, relaxing in the pose (if you do not wish to continue further, then release slowly and repeat this much on the other side).

b, c) The following reclining variations of the hero pose deepen the stretch. Start by placing the hands on the floor behind you. Raise the left knee and place the sole of the foot on the floor in front of the sitting bone. Keep the right leg folded alongside the hip. Lean back and momentarily lift the pelvis to draw the tailbone under and lengthen the lower back while pressing the right knee down. Then lower the pelvis to the floor and lean back on the elbows. There should be no strain in the knees. Finally, come all the way onto the back, again adjusting the pelvis and lower back, and lengthening through the top of the thigh. Rest your hands at your abdomen, center yourself, and breathe in the pose. When you are ready to come out, raise your torso by supporting it with the arms. Repeat on the other side.

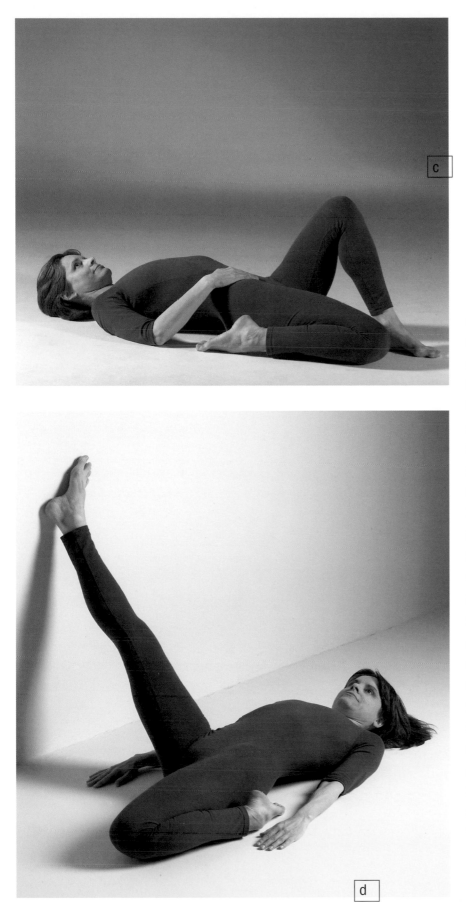

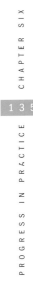

d) You can deepen the work in the reclining pose by placing one foot on the wall, allowing you to press the pelvis down and open the thigh. Sit with your right hip and shoulder a few feet away from a wall; then bring the top of the left foot alongside the hip, rest the right foot on the floor with the knee raised, and lower into the reclining posture just as you did before. Next, straighten the right leg and place the right foot on the wall, pressing it gently into the wall. Press the left knee into the floor and lengthen the thigh. Walk the foot up or down the wall or closer to the head to explore the stretch in the thigh and pelvis. Reposition yourself closer or further to the wall as needed to make the stretch more effective and comfortable. To come out of the pose, lower the right foot to the floor and slowly return to a sitting position. Then repeat on the other side.

Easy Pose Forward Bend

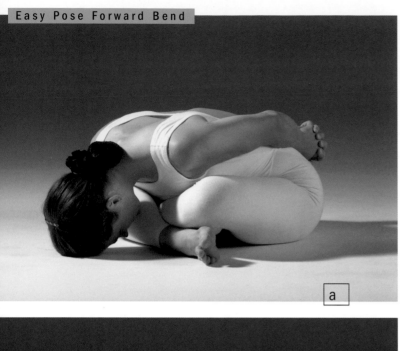

a

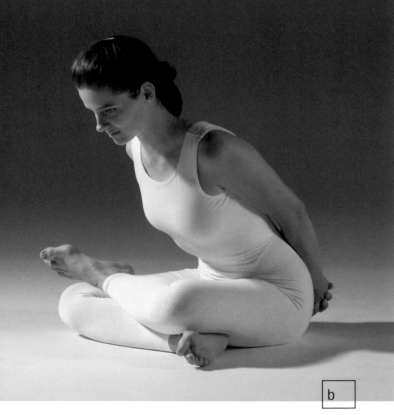

b

Easy Pose Forward Bend

This simple forward bend stretches the piriformis muscle and other external hip rotators. These muscles are often tight and may contribute to restrictions in hip mobility as well as to sciatic nerve pain. The pose also stretches muscles of the back and spine all the way to the base of the skull.

a) Sit on the floor with your legs crossed in the easy pose (or sit on a cushion to support the lower back). Clasp your hands behind your back and lengthen your spine up through the crown of the head. Grounding the pelvis on the floor, bend forward from the hips and extend the chest out and over the legs. Continue to bend forward, keeping the back flat as long as possible before releasing the abdomen, the shoulders, and finally the head toward the floor. The arms may be brought to the floor in front, or they may remain at the back. Center and breathe in the pose. As you inhale let the back expand, and as you exhale release further toward the floor. To come out of the pose lift the head, the shoulders, and finally the lower back, returning to an upright position.

b) To deepen the stretch, reposition the legs. Bend the right knee and place the lower right leg on the floor in front of you. Then place the lower left leg on the right leg so that the left knee rests above the right foot, and the outside left ankle rests on the right calf or knee. Adjust the two legs until they are stable, ground the pelvis, and extend up through the length of the spine. Then clasp the hands behind the back and bend forward as before. (Once down, keep the hands at the back or release them to the front.) Notice that as you deepen the forward bend in this and the previous posture the pubic bones tilt forward and toward the floor, the sacrum moves back and away from the floor, and the abdomen is pressed toward the legs. Relax and center in the pose; then repeat on the opposite side.

Reclining Hip Stretch

This passive stretch improves the range of movement at the hip and stretches the hamstrings and adductor muscles of the inner thigh.

a) Lie on your back, bending the knees and raising them toward the chest. Reach around the outside of the legs and grasp the instep of each foot with the hands. Lift the feet until the soles face the ceiling and the shins are perpendicular to the floor. Then pull firmly on the feet and press the knees toward the floor on either side of the torso. As the knees are drawn down, press the lower back and sacrum toward the floor as well. Keep the spine long, and relax deeply in the hip joints.

b) To deepen the stretch, shift your grip to the toes (or hold the calves or thighs with your hands). Now slowly straighten the knees and open the legs out to the side, drawing the feet apart with your hands. Again, press the lower back and sacrum toward the floor. Hold for 5–10 breaths, relaxing resistance in the inner thighs. Then bring the legs together, bend the knees, and release from the pose.

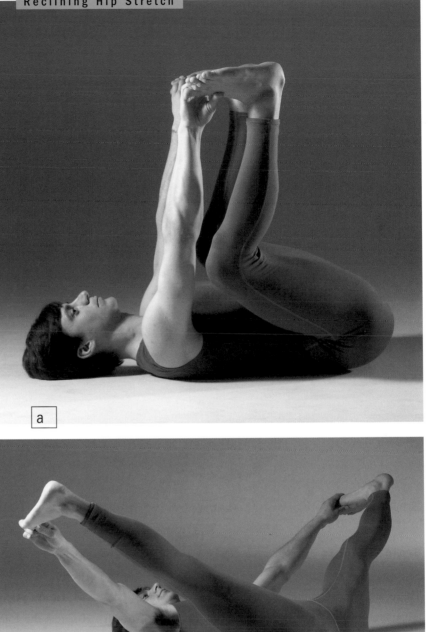

a

b

Groin Openers

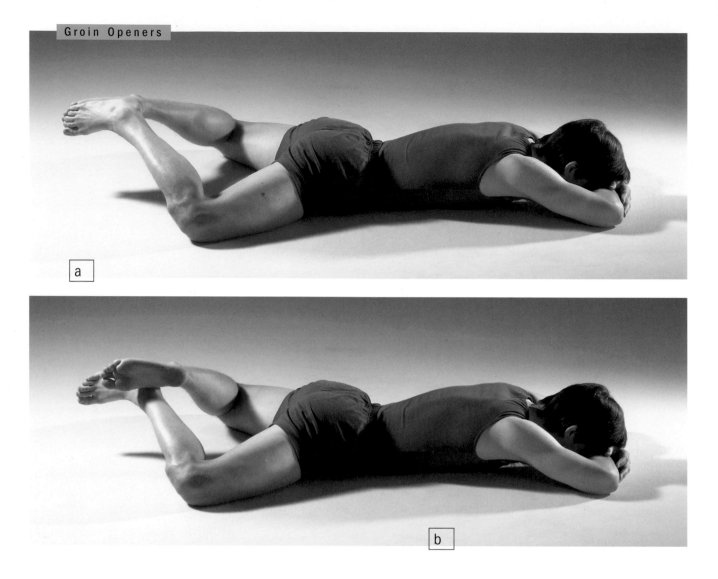

a

b

138

Groin Openers

These are intense stretches for everyone. They take advantage of gravity and the weight of the legs to stretch the inner thighs and groin, so relax and release the weight of the pelvis to the floor in all the variations.

a) Lie on your stomach with your chin on the floor (or rest the forehead on the crossed forearms). Bend the knees and spread them as far apart as possible; then bring the soles of the feet together. Without lifting the pelvis or changing the placement of the knees, relax the inner thighs and the muscles around the hip joints. Let the feet lower toward the floor, but keep the soles of the feet together. Relax deeply into the pose and breathe, allowing the weight of the legs to gently open the inner thighs and groin.

b) Next, increase the bend at the knees slightly and cross one ankle above the other. Again, relax the tension in the hip joint, groin, and pelvis. Notice how the stretch intensifies. Then cross the ankles in the other direction. Hold each side until you feel ready to release.

c) Finally, with the soles of the feet together once again, place the hands on the floor under the shoulders. Lift the head and chest as in the cobra pose (p.94). Then slowly straighten the arms and continue to arch upward, lengthening the spine and stretching the front of the torso. Keep the shoulders and shoulder blades down and the soles of the feet pressed together. The pelvis is suspended between the knees. Release in the groin on each side, softening and allowing gravity to gently open the pelvis and draw it toward the floor. Hold the pose, relaxing resistance and breathing smoothly; then bend the arms and slowly return to the floor when you are ready to release.

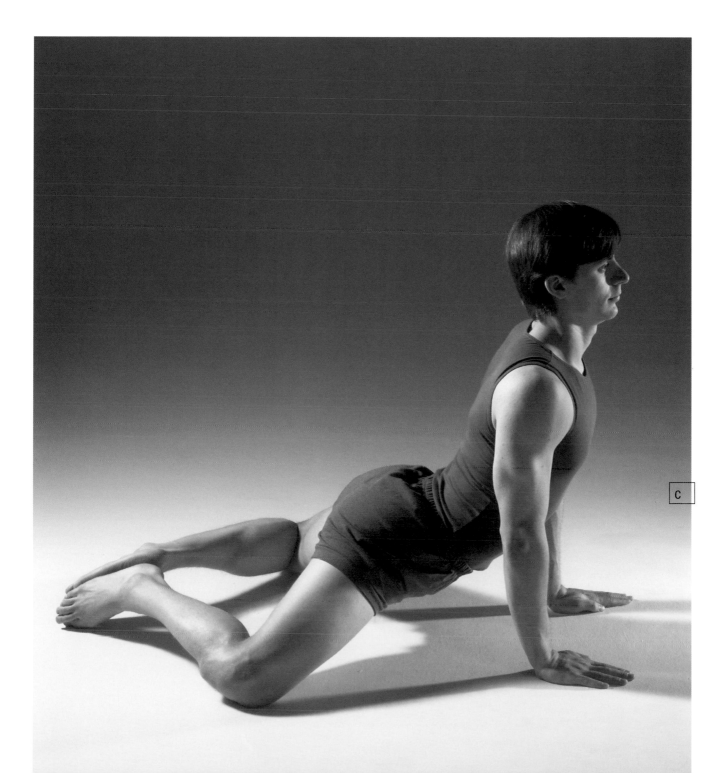

C

Frog Pose

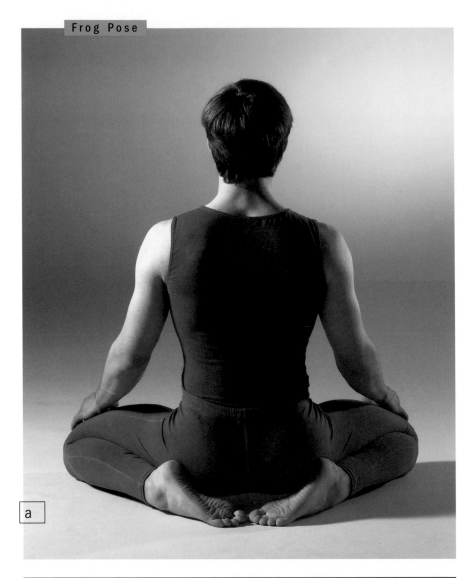

a

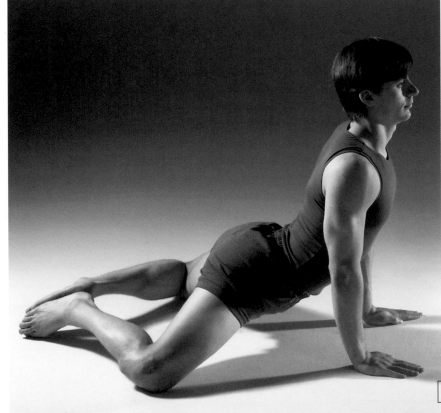

b

Frog Pose (Mandukasana)

a) The frog pose stretches the quadriceps as well as the muscles in the inner thigh and groin. You can move into the groin openers from this pose as well. Begin by sitting between the heels with the knees open to the sides and the big toes touching (if necessary, use cushions to support the hips and reduce strain at the knees). Lengthen the spine up out of the pelvis through the crown of the head. Center yourself and breathe smoothly, gradually stretching the inner thigh and groin on each side, and allowing the sitting bones to release toward the floor.

b) Next, keeping the lower legs in place, lift the pelvis and lean forward, placing your hands on the floor. Walk the hands away from the legs, bring the soles of the feet together, and press the pelvis forward and down until you are in the upward-facing groin opener (the previous sequence). As before, roll the shoulders down and back, lift the head and neck up out of the shoulders, lift the sternum, and arch the spine as the pelvis releases toward the floor. Hold and breathe, relaxing the groin areas, inner thighs, and lower abdomen. To release, slowly lift the pelvis, walk the hands back toward the legs, and return to the frog pose. Then bring the knees together and sit off to the side.

Butterfly Pose and Variations (Baddha Konasana)

The combination of hip opening and forward bending accomplished in these poses stretches the inner thighs, the hamstrings, and the hip rotators (which can be felt deep in the buttocks). The lower back must remain strong. Keep your awareness circulating through the pelvis and inner thighs, and pay special attention to relaxing tension in the hip joints.

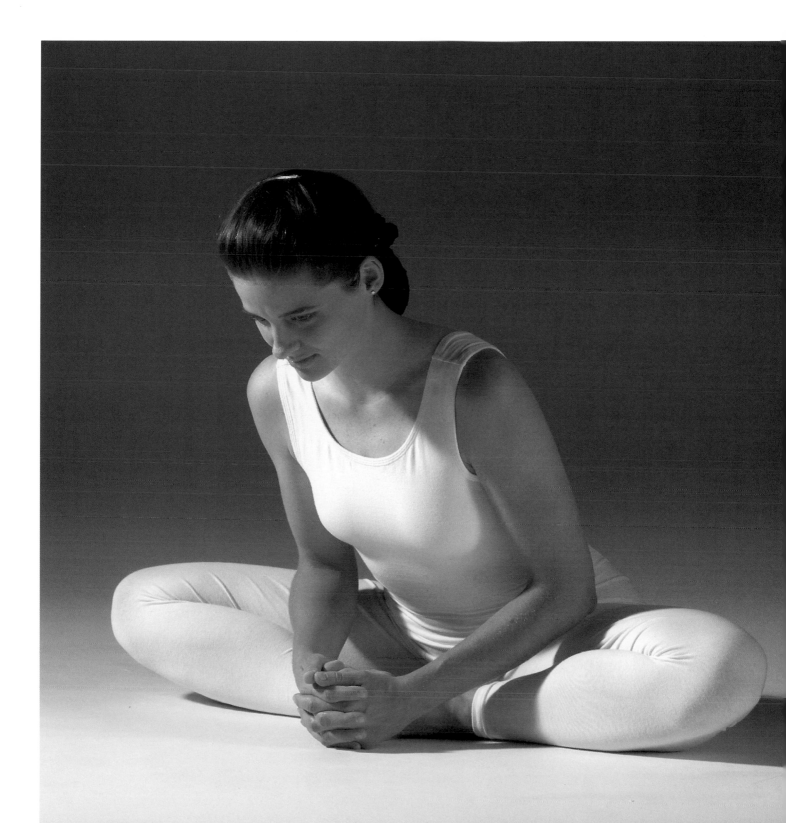

a) Sit on the floor (or on a cushion, to keep the lower back from rounding). Bring the soles of the feet together and draw the heels toward the pelvis. Grasping the feet with the hands, open the knees and press them toward the floor. Then lift the lower back and lengthen through the crown of the head, resting firmly on the sitting bones. Center yourself in the pose and breathe smoothly, gradually relaxing resistance and lowering the knees further toward the floor.

b) To deepen the stretch, lift the lower back and keep it straight as you bend forward from the hips, shifting your weight toward the front of the sitting bones and pressing the abdomen forward and then down toward the feet and inner thighs. If you are very flexible you may be able to lower your head onto the floor; otherwise, center yourself in the stretch that is comfortable for you and breathe deeply into the abdomen and the sides of the rib cage.

Butterfly Pose and Variations

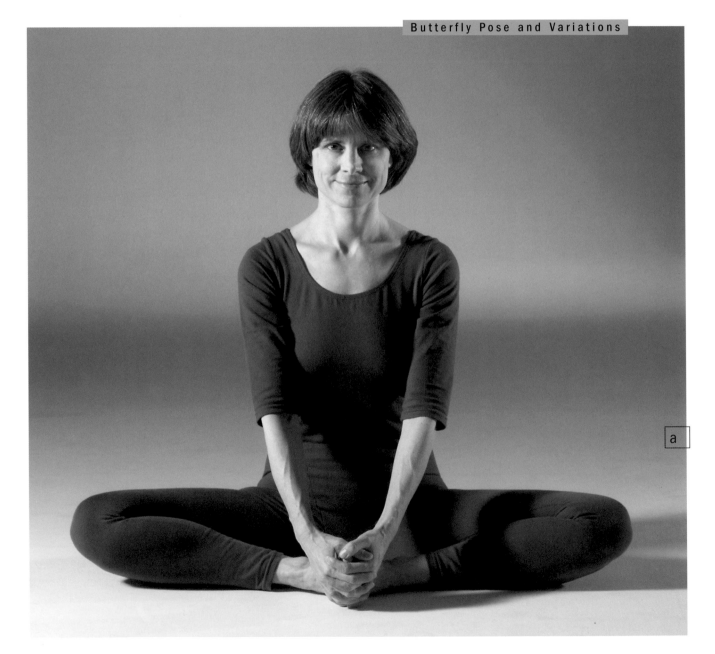

a

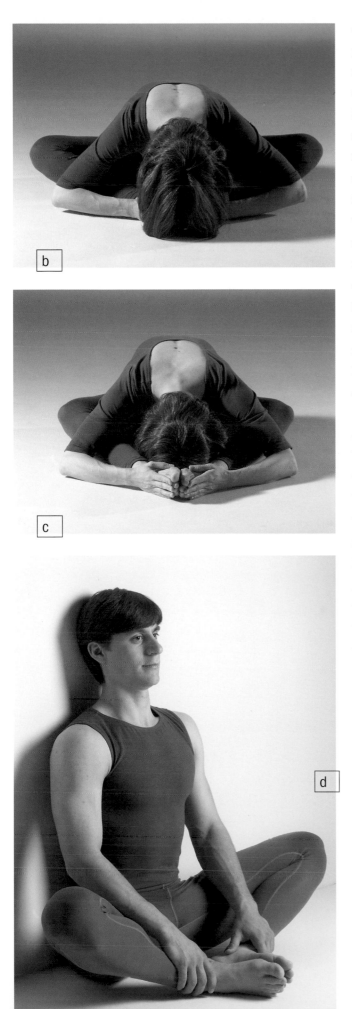

b

c

d

c) To explore the forward bend and the stretch it provides for the back, legs, and buttocks, return the torso to the center and move the feet 6–8 inches farther away from the pelvis. Next, grasping the feet with the hands, extend forward once again, lengthening the spine and bending from the hips. Keep the soles of the feet together as you hold and breathe. Then lift the torso and repeat the process in a series of steps, moving the feet an additional few inches away and bending forward with each successive step. Notice how the stretch is altered as the placement of the feet changes. Finally, move the feet as far forward as you can with the soles still pressed together. Bring the face toward the floor behind the heels (if you are very flexible, then rest your forehead on the floor). Center yourself in whatever bend is most comfortable for you, and breathe smoothly. Then lift the head, the shoulders, and the lower back, releasing out of the pose.

d) The butterfly pose is difficult for many students because of tightness in the inner thighs. A good way to stretch these muscles is to sit on the floor with your back against a wall. Keep the back of the pelvis and the base of the spine as close to the wall as you can, and lengthen through the crown of the head. Bend the knees, clasp the hands around the feet, and release the knees toward the floor. Then use the palms of the hands to firmly massage the inner thighs from the groin toward the knee. Finally, within your capacity, carefully press the thighs and knees further toward the floor with your hands. Hold the pose and breathe smoothly and evenly, as if the breath is flowing into the whole body. If you like, you may also bend forward from the hips, further deepening the stretch.

Seated Angle Pose (Upavishta Konasana)

The seated angle pose is similar to the butterfly posture. It also stretches the adductor muscles of the inner thighs and the hamstrings, and opens the back of the legs and the lower back.

a) Begin by sitting on the floor with the legs straight out in front (if helpful, place a cushion under the pelvis to keep the lower back from rounding). Spread the legs apart, keeping them straight and equidistant from the center line of the torso. The knees and toes point straight up, and the back of the knees are pressed toward the floor. With the hands behind the hips on either side, raise the pelvis off the floor momentarily. Spread the legs a bit further apart, aligning the pelvis and lifting the lower back. Then lower the pelvis back to the floor and sit firmly on the sitting bones with the hands resting on the legs.

b) Next, bring the hands onto the floor between the legs. Lift the lower back and bend forward from the hips, walking the hands to the front. As the torso extends forward, keep the toes and kneecaps pointing straight up. Hold at whatever point you are able, breathing and centering yourself in the pose. Soften the abdomen and stretch the back of the legs all the way to the heels while maintaining a firm lower back. Feel the sacrum being lifted by the forward tilt of the pelvis while the pubic bones are drawn down between the thighs. Hold for a number of breaths, relaxing resistance and deepening into the pose. Then slowly release and bring the legs together.

Seated Angle Pose

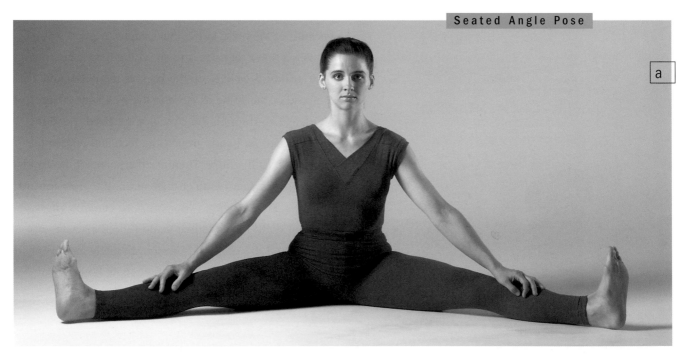

a

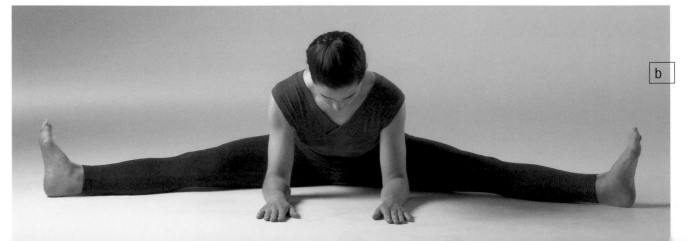

b

Inner Thigh Stretch on the Wall

This stretch is similar to the seated angle pose, but it works particularly well for those who are stiff in the lower back and inner thighs and have trouble sitting up straight with their legs open to the sides. With the spine and lower back supported on the floor, gravity works to open the legs and gently stretch the adductor muscles.

a) Begin by sitting on the floor with the outside of one hip and shoulder against the wall, and your hands behind you on the floor.

b) To come into the pose lean back, bringing the knees to the chest and lifting the feet. Then rotate the body so that you are lying down on your back with the tailbone near the wall and the top of the head pointed away from it. Extend the legs vertically against the wall and rest the back on the floor. Support the head and neck by interlacing the fingers behind the head and opening the elbows. Then spread the legs out to the sides, keeping them supported by the wall. Relax and allow gravity to draw the legs down and stretch the inside of the thighs. Avoid strain in the back of the knees; bend the knees slightly if you feel discomfort there. To make the stretch more active, lengthen the spine and press the tailbone to the wall; lengthen through the back of the legs and press the heels away from the pelvis; keep the knees and heels firmly against the wall without rotating the legs in either direction. Breathe as you center yourself in the pose, gradually increasing the holding time over a number of practice sessions and relaxing more deeply.

Release the pose by bringing the legs back together on the wall, bending the knees toward the chest, and sliding the soles of the feet down the wall. Relax, resting the legs and lower back and relieving tension on the inside of the knees. Finally, roll to one side and come out of the pose.

Inner Thigh Stretch on the Wall

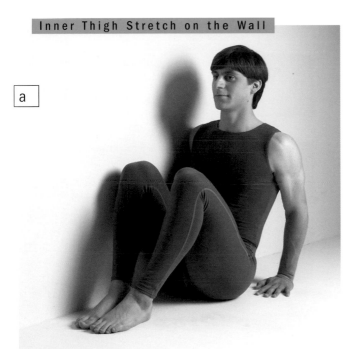

a

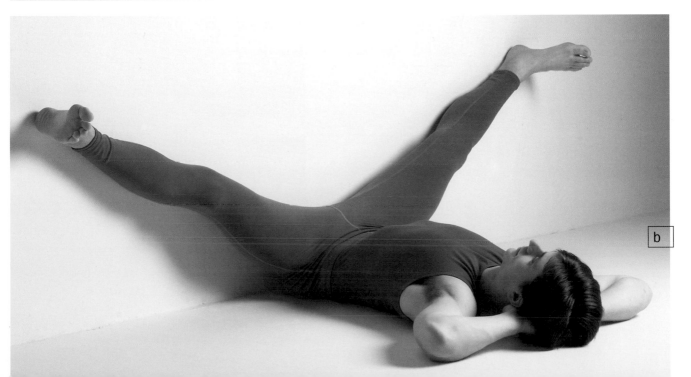

b

TIGHT HAMSTRINGS

Tight hamstrings are the bane of many aspiring students because they restrict some of the most important movements in hatha yoga. These muscles originate from the sitting bones in the pelvis; they extend down the back of the thighs and attach just below the knees. In a standing position, if you bend forward from the hip joints while keeping the knees straight and the back flat, you will stretch these muscles. If they are tight, however, the lower back often rounds to compensate. Tight hamstrings can also cause chronic problems with pelvic and spinal alignment, leading to weakness and pain in the back.

The hamstrings work in coordination with the quadriceps, the muscles on the front of the thighs. If the hamstrings are tight, then include asanas that activate and strengthen the quadriceps as part of your regular routine. Also, while stretching the hamstrings, experiment with pulling the kneecaps up and tightening the quadriceps to encourage the hamstrings to lengthen more easily. The following stretches from Asana Sequences One and Two focus on the hamstrings and will prepare you for the more difficult hamstring stretches to follow:

Standing forward stretches pp.30, 31

Couch pose p.40

Seated forward stretch p.41

Triangle pose p.79

Angle pose p.82

Standing spread-legged forward bend p.84

Head-to-knee pose p.103

Sun salutation p.70

Muscles of the Hip and Thigh

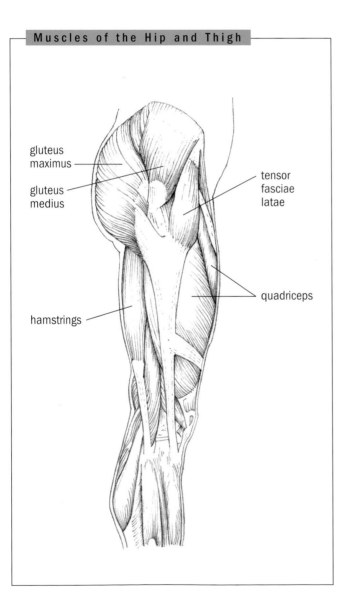

gluteus maximus

gluteus medius

tensor fasciae latae

quadriceps

hamstrings

Strap Stretch on the Back

This is an excellent stretch for those with a limited range of movement as well as for more flexible students, because in this pose the lower back is supported by the floor and the stretch is concentrated in the back of the leg.

a) Lie on your back. Bend the right knee toward the chest and wrap a strap (a belt or an old necktie work well) around the ball of the foot.

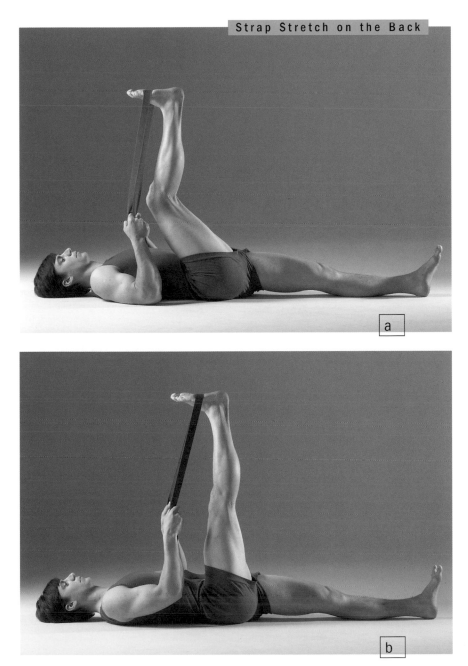

Strap Stretch on the Back

a

b

b) Slowly straighten the knee. Activate the quadriceps, pulling the kneecap up, and lengthening through the heel. As you straighten the leg, keep the back of the shoulders on the floor and do not round the lower back. Hold and breathe, relaxing and lengthening through the back of the right leg. To deepen the stretch draw the foot further overhead, keeping the leg straight. Anchor the pelvis and lengthen the lower leg, maintaining firm contact with the floor. Another option is to bend the lower leg, pressing the sole of the foot into the floor and grounding the lower back. In any case, if you experience discomfort behind the knee, or if the knee hyperextends, bend it slightly and shift the stretch to the back of the thigh. Center yourself in the pose, relaxing resistance and deepening the stretch. Then release and repeat on the opposite side.

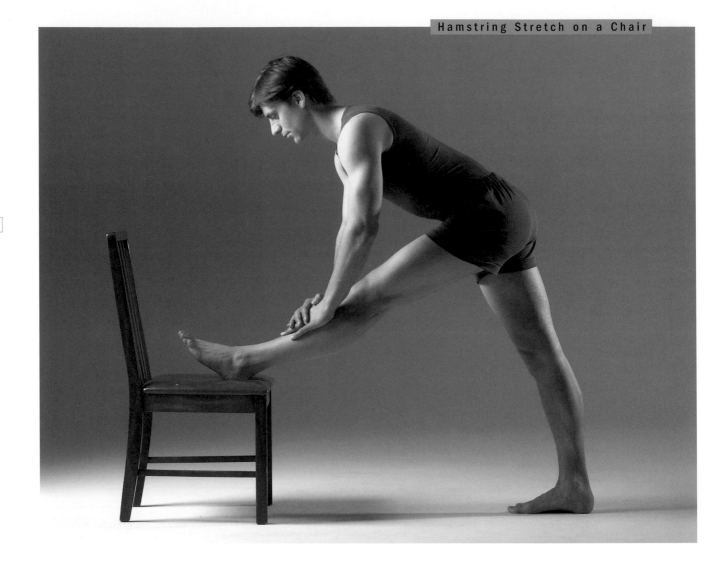

Hamstring Stretch on a Chair

This is an easy, effective stretch that you can do almost anywhere, anytime.

Place the left heel on a chair and straighten the left leg, resting the hands on the thigh. Keep the spine long and the right foot firm and pointed straight ahead on the floor. Lift the kneecaps, activating the quadriceps in both legs. There should be no strain behind the knees. Now bend forward from the hips, taking care not to round the lower back. Walk the hands down the leg (keep the leg straight) until you have stretched to your comfortable capacity. Hold and breathe, relaxing resistance. Throughout the stretch keep the upper back erect and the shoulders moving down away from the ears. Increase the holding time gradually without straining the knee. Release slowly and repeat the stretch on the other side.

Standing Forward Bend Variations (Uttanasana)

The standing forward bends open and stretch the back as well as the back of the legs. They are also calming and quieting to the mind.

a) Stand with your feet hip-width apart and place the palms of your hands on your buttocks. Maintaining a flat lower back, exhale and bend forward from the hip joints, sliding the hands down the back of the thighs. Then bend the knees, and again exhaling, use the arms to help fold the torso down onto the thighs (still keeping the back flat and the head in line). Hold and breathe.

b) Next, lower the head and neck, and slide the hands further down the legs to the calves or ankles. Using the arms to keep the torso as close as possible to the legs, slowly straighten the knees, tilting the pelvis forward and raising the sitting bones. Do not strain the lower back. Center your weight, pressing down equally on the balls of the feet and the heels. Then hold and breathe, centering in the stretch.

c) Release the hands from the legs and fold the arms, suspending them from the shoulders. As a result, the torso will move slightly farther away from the legs. Activate the quadriceps, pulling the kneecaps up and lengthening through the back of the legs. Tilt the pelvis forward, raising and spreading the sitting bones and lengthening the lower back. To deepen the posture try bending and then straightening the knees, using the temporary release in the hamstrings to extend the downward stretch in the lower back.

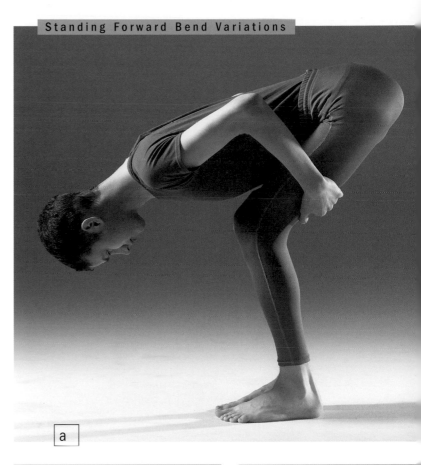

a

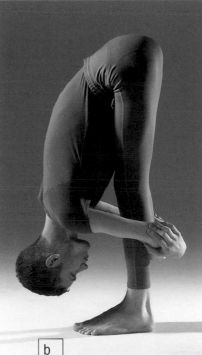

b

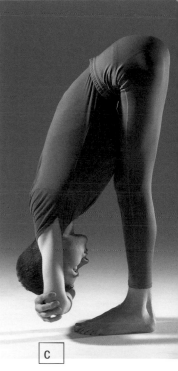

c

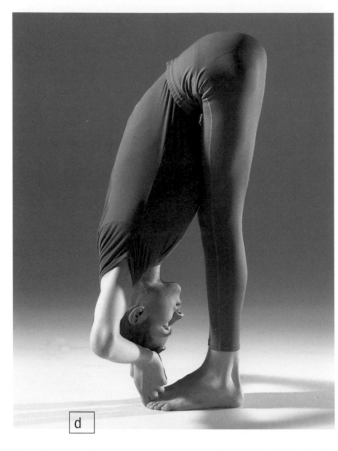

d

d) Finally, grasp the back of the legs, the ankles, or the large toes with the hands, and once more gently draw the torso closer to the legs. Hold and breathe, centering yourself in the pose. When you are ready to come out of the posture, bend the knees and lift the head, the neck, and the upper torso. Then flatten the lower back and slowly return to a standing pose. To release back strain you may wish to follow this pose with the child's pose (p.34) or with a gentle backward-bending pose such as the arch (p.118).

e) The standing forward bends may be challenging for the back. If so, try using a chair for support as you bend forward. Stand far enough away from the chair to keep the arms and torso extended and the legs straight. Hold on to the chair to support your weight, and to gently lengthen the spine as you stretch forward and down. Pull the kneecaps up as before, tilting the pelvis forward and lifting the sitting bones. Concentrate on the back of the legs, and be gentle with the back.

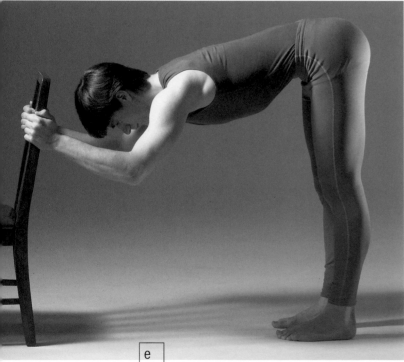

e

Head-to-Knee Pose— Crossed-Leg Variation

In this variation the added weight of the leg resting on the thigh intensifies the stretch by pressing the back of the thigh into the floor.

Sit with the legs straight out in front (use a cushion, if necessary, to prevent the lower back from rounding). Bend the right knee and place the right ankle on the left thigh just above the knee (the ankle-bone crosses the thigh). Open the right hip and lower the knee parallel to the floor. Ground the sitting bones and lift the lower back, stretching through the back of the left leg. Exhaling, bend forward from the hips, further elongating the spine as you extend out and over the left leg. Do not strain either knee. The hands can remain on the folded right leg, or slide out toward the left foot. Hold the pose and breathe smoothly and evenly, centering in the stretch. As you relax, deepen the stretch by bending further forward. When you are ready, release slowly and come back to an upright posture. Then repeat on the other side.

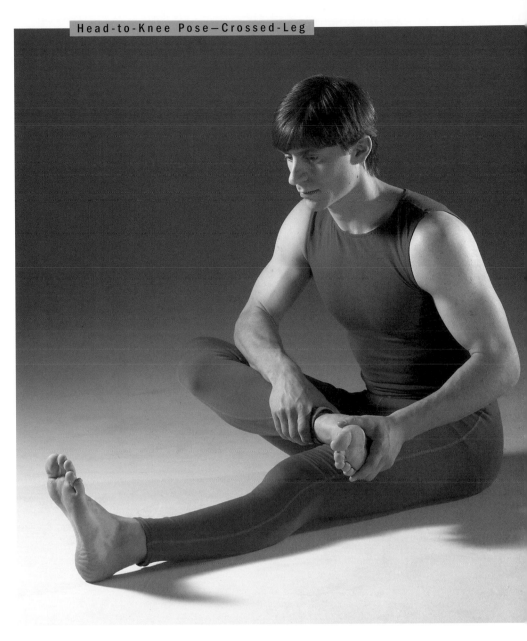

Deep Back Muscles

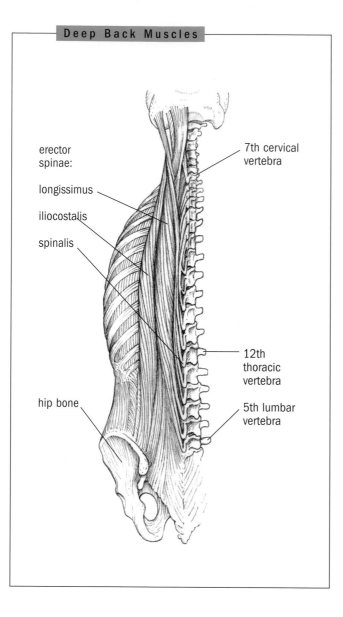

erector
spine:

longissimus

iliocostalis

spinalis

hip bone

7th cervical
vertebra

12th
thoracic
vertebra

5th lumbar
vertebra

LOWER BACK

The lower back is a crossroads for muscles that run from the pelvis and thighs below to the upper back and head above. These muscles also span the space between the twelfth rib and the pelvis, stabilize and mobilize the lower back, protect the abdominal organs, moderate and control forward bending, and assist in backward and side bending. The outermost layers of the deep spinal muscles run from the pelvis to the neck, deeper layers connect multiple segments of the spine, and the deepest layers join neighboring vertebrae.

Spinal muscles are sensitive to emotional tension, and frequently such tension is punctuated by lower back pain. A balanced selection of yoga postures will develop both strength and flexibility in the back, preserving your ability to twist, bend, elongate, and rotate the spine. Equally important, a healthy lower back provides the foundation for good posture.

Many lower back problems result from misalignments caused by muscular imbalances in the hips, legs, and abdomen, and these regions all need to be addressed in any therapeutic program for lower back problems, but the spinal muscles that run from the neck to the pelvis need special attention. Many postures exercise the deep back muscles, especially the cobra and locust poses, the cat stretch, and the staff pose. And to help release tension in the lower back, several exercises in Asana Sequences One and Two are invaluable. The postures and exercises listed on this page stabilize the pelvis and lower back by strengthening and stretching muscles of the thighs, pelvis, abdomen, and upper back. Pay special attention to:

 Reclining twists pp.22, 92, 117

 Cat pose p.32

 Rock around the clock p.38

 Inside twist p.39

 Knees-to-chest pose pp.45, 49

 Child's pose p.89

 Staff pose p.102

 Hip-balancing sequence p.109

 Pelvic tilt and arch pp.46, 118

 Lunge pose p.35

 Flat-back forward bends pp.30, 84

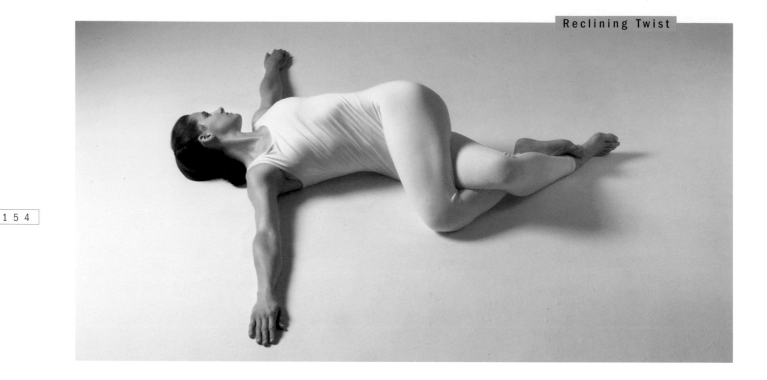

Additional Help for the Lower Back

Reclining Twist

The reclining twists stretch the whole spine, but they are particularly effective for stretching the muscles of the lower back. There are many different variations; this one emphasizes the legs, inner thighs, and lower spine.

Lie on your back, knees bent and feet on the floor near the pelvis. The arms are extended from the shoulders, palms down. Cross the left thigh over the right, wrapping the legs tightly (if possible, catch the right shin with the toes of the left foot). Now lift the pelvis off the floor momentarily, sliding the right hip underneath and toward the center. Then lower the pelvis, twist to the right, and let the wrapped legs release toward the floor.

If you are very flexible you may be able to keep both the legs and the left arm and shoulder on the floor at the same time. For most, however, the pose evolves over many practice sessions by alternately working with the twist in the lower torso (keeping the shoulder and arm firmly anchored) and then the twist in the upper torso (allowing the shoulder and arm to initially release from the floor, and then drawing them back). Whichever alternative you have chosen, breathe deeply into the abdomen as you center yourself in the pose. When you are ready, return to the center and repeat on the other side.

Locust Pose Variations
(Shalabhasana)

Muscle tone, strength, and flexibility are seldom equal on both sides of the body, and this is as true for the pelvis and lower back as it is for the arms and legs. These variations of the locust pose help restore muscular balance deep in the pelvis and realign the sacroiliac joint. They strengthen the muscles of the lower back and buttocks; they may provide quick relief to simple lower back discomfort, as well as prevent lower back problems from developing.

a) Lie on your stomach with the chin on the floor and the legs together. The arms are alongside the body, palms down. Bend the right knee and flex the ankle so that the sole of the foot faces up. Exhaling, lift the right thigh and press the foot toward the ceiling. Once the leg is raised, turn your attention to the left side of the body, relaxing the lower back, the buttock, and the leg, and grounding the pelvis. This will isolate muscle contractions on the right, and you may not be able to lift the leg as high as before. For maximum benefit in this pose, adjust to the new height and carefully observe the contrast between the two sides of your body as you breathe out and in. Finally, release the right leg, noting any residual tension on the left side. Relax for 3 breaths and repeat on the other side.

b) Now bend both knees. Tighten the buttocks and press the lower abdomen into the floor. Exhaling, lift both thighs equidistant from the floor, keeping the chin down and the feet square. Keep the knees directly in line with the hips. Stretch up equally through the inner and outer edges of the feet, and out through the toes. Hold for 3 breaths, then gently release back to the floor. Repeat 2 more times. Watch your feet in a mirror, or have a friend watch you, correcting tendencies to rotate the toes out, lift one foot higher than the other, or tilt the feet.

Locust Pose Variations

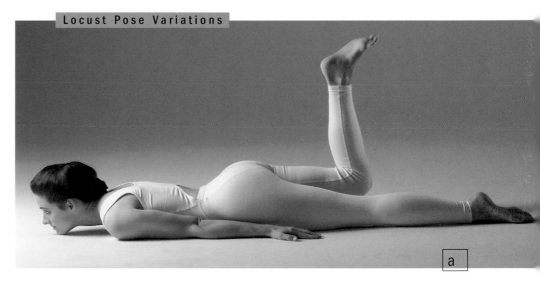

a

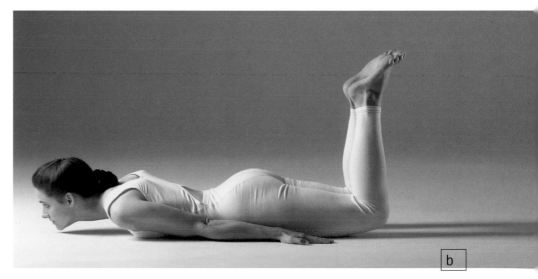

b

Squat Pose with Variations

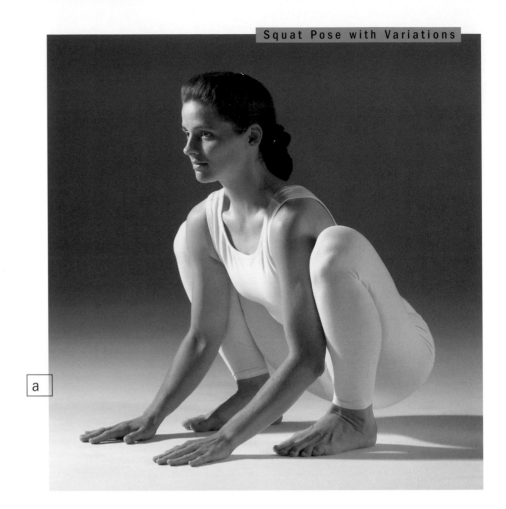

a

Squat Pose with Variations

Squatting poses are excellent for stretching and releasing tension in the lower back, developing elasticity in the ankles and knees, relieving tired legs, increasing flexibility in the hips, and massaging the abdominal organs.

a) Stand with the feet parallel and just wider than hip-width apart (this distance between the feet makes the pose easier, while narrowing the distance makes the pose more difficult). Bend the knees and lower the pelvis toward the floor into a squatting pose. Allow the heels to come off the floor if necessary to keep your balance, but maintain the alignment of the feet. If your knees feel strained, check your foot alignment again or redistribute your weight. Drop down through the heels and the tailbone, while at the same time stretching the torso up and forward. If you have come all the way down with the heels remaining on the floor, then spread the knees and place the hands on the floor, arms between the legs. Hold and breathe.

b) If you are uncomfortable, or if the heels don't reach the floor, try either of the following modifications. Start by placing a firm folded blanket or mat under the heels. Lower the heels onto the support and open the knees, keeping the feet pointed straight ahead. Folding at the hip joints while broadening and flattening the lower back, extend the torso forward between the thighs. Then hold and breathe, relaxing more deeply into the pose. A second method for lowering the heels in the pose is to spread the knees and hold on to a stable support (a low ledge, railing, or piece of heavy furniture will do). Use the support to counter falling backward as you lower the heels further toward the floor. Once in the pose, lengthen and flatten the spine and lower the torso between the legs, continuing to use the support to maintain the pose. Hold and breathe.

c) If you can bring the soles of the feet flat to the floor, then the next challenge is to gradually bring the feet together. At any point in the process it may help you to momentarily lift onto the balls of the feet, open the thighs, and press the torso forward and down. Then release the heels back to the floor again. Once you can bring the armpits inside the knees, spread the elbows to the sides and grasp the outer ankles with the hands. If possible, lower the head and the tailbone toward the floor.

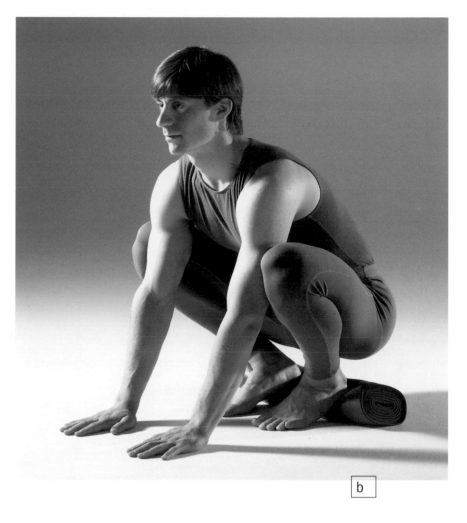

b

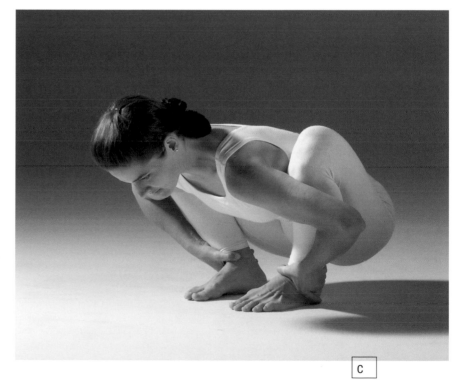

c

WEAK ABDOMEN AND HIP FLEXORS

Three layers of muscles encircle the abdomen like a corset, running from front to back and from the rib cage to the pelvis. They compress the abdomen during defecation, during childbirth, and sometimes during breathing. They support and protect the abdominal organs, and they also preserve good posture by resisting an exaggerated arching in the lower back. Encased within these layers in the front are two parallel bands of muscle that extend from the pubic bones upward to the sternum. These strong muscles are important flexors of the spine; they fold it forward. In addition, as we have already seen, the iliopsoas muscles flex the hips.

Strong and flexible abdominal muscles are the foundation of a fruitful yoga practice. Toning the abdominal muscles and organs also brings myriad other benefits, such as improved digestion and elimination, freedom from lower back pain, relief from cramps and other menstrual problems, and improved overall energy and enthusiasm. Many different exercises are helpful for working with the abdominal muscles and hip flexors. Leglifts strengthen the hip flexors, which form a vital link between the thighs below and the torso above; curls target the abdominal muscles. You need to do both. Agni sara (p.188), the fire series (pp.90, 159), and related practices not only tone all the abdominal muscles but also awaken the vital energy which enlivens us both physically and mentally. To prepare yourself for further work on the hip flexors and abdominal muscles, concentrate on:

 Abdominal squeeze p.30

 Hip-balancing sequence p.109

 Curls p.38

 Beginning fire series p.90

 Sun salutation p.70

Abdominal Muscles

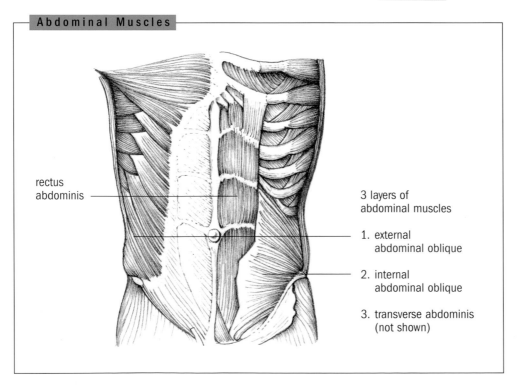

rectus abdominis

3 layers of abdominal muscles

1. external abdominal oblique

2. internal abdominal oblique

3. transverse abdominis (not shown)

Additional Work for
Abdominal Strength

The Advanced Fire Series

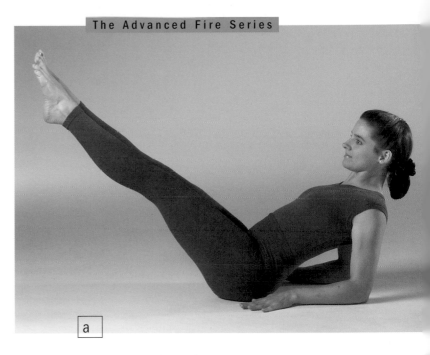

The fire series is a set of seven different leglifts, varying in difficulty and performed with the weight of the upper torso supported on the elbows. Throughout these variations it is important to work within your capacity, challenging your body without straining it. If the lower back begins to ache or feel weak either while in the postures or afterwards, switch to an easier version of the pose or come out of the pose altogether and rest. A few repetitions daily will benefit you much more than the occasional long session, and regular practice is the key to developing strength.

To come into the basic position, sit on the floor with the legs extended in front of you. Lean back and place the elbows on the floor under the shoulders, the forearms parallel to the sides of the body. Press down through the arms to open the chest and straighten the spine while lengthening through the crown of the head. Pull the shoulders away from the ears, and keep the chin drawn toward the throat. The face and jaw are relaxed and the breath is full and deep. Focus on the navel center.

a) *Double leglift.* Inhaling, lift both legs halfway up—to 45 degrees. Then exhaling, lower them to just above the floor. Raise and lower the legs slowly, repeating 5 or more times.

b) *Double leglift, continued.* Inhaling, lift both legs slowly to 90 degrees, lower slowly to 20 degrees, then lift back to 90 degrees. Continue for 5 repetitions, inhaling up and exhaling down.

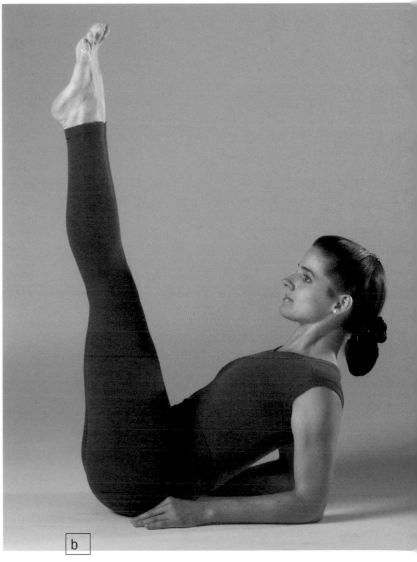

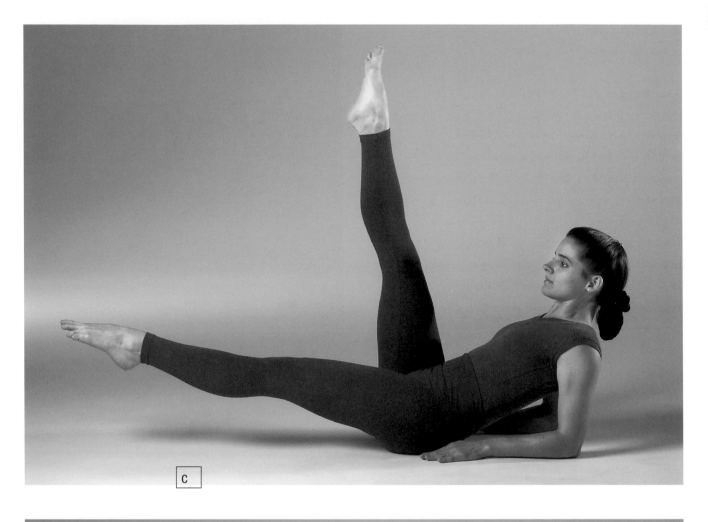

c

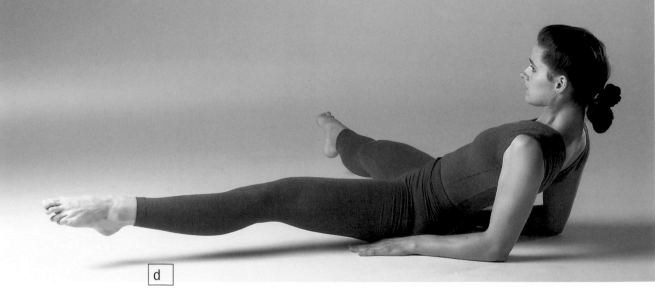

d

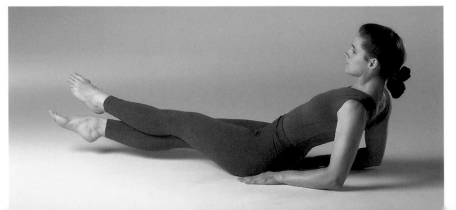

c) *Vertical scissors*. The legs cross in midair as you lift one to 90 degrees while lowering the other just above the floor. Move slowly, keeping the legs straight and the toes reaching out.

d) *Lateral scissors*. Lift the legs to about 20 degrees, then open them to the sides and cross one leg over the other as you bring the legs together. Repeat 3–5 times, alternating the top leg.

e) *Bicycle*. Keep the legs about 20 degrees off the floor. Draw alternate knees to the chest as you push out through the foot of the other leg. Consciously press one thigh to the abdomen at the same time that you push the opposite foot away from the body. Work for a push-pull, piston-like feeling. Repeat 5 or more times.

f) *Split-leg circling*. Lift both legs to 90 degrees, then open them out to the side and circle down to about 20 degrees. Bring them together, still off the floor, and lift back to 90 degrees. Continue circling 5 times. Move slowly, and feel the rotation in the hip joint and the action of the inner thighs.

   Reverse variation. Lift both legs to 20 degrees, open them out to the side, circle them out and up to 90 degrees, and bring them together at 90 degrees. Lower to 20 degrees and continue for 5 repetitions.

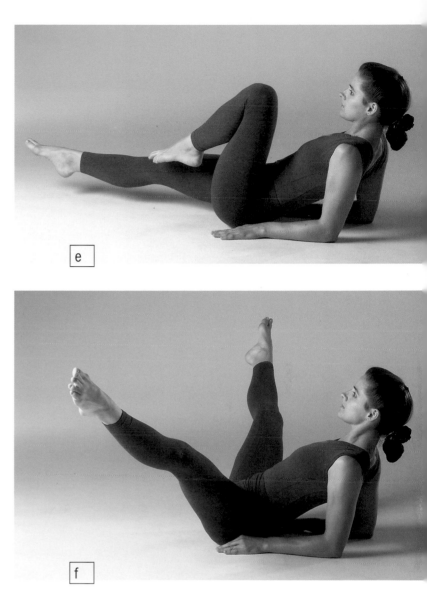

e

f

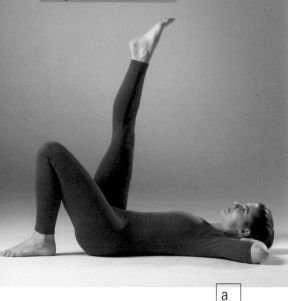

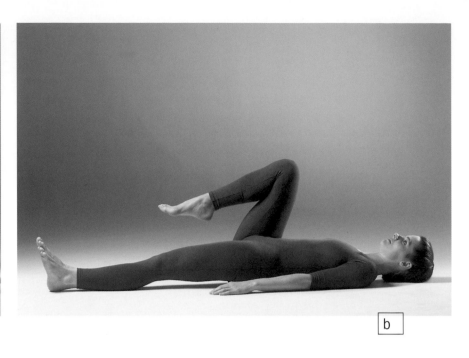

Leglift Variations

a

b

Leglift Variations

The primary difference between these leglift variations and the fire series is that here the back is resting firmly on the floor. A number of different arm positions are possible. The arms offer the most support when they are alongside the body or even slightly under the lower back. For more challenge, interlace the fingers behind the head and open the elbows to the floor. This opens the upper chest and helps keep the head, neck, and shoulders relaxed and stable. For the most challenge, bring the arms onto the floor overhead.

Avoid pain or strain in all leglifts. First practice the variations you can perform comfortably, gradually increasing the number of repetitions before adding variations of greater difficulty. As you lift the legs, use your abdominal muscles to stabilize the pelvis by pressing the lower back toward the floor. Keep the shoulders and upper back completely stationary and relaxed. Soften the face and jaw, breathing smoothly and cultivating a feeling of ease. The following variations are progressively more difficult.

a) *Single leglifts, bent knees.* Lie on your back with the knees raised and feet on the floor near the pelvis. Cradle your head in your hands with the elbows open to the sides. Inhaling, lift one knee, then straighten the leg and extend it toward the ceiling. Exhaling, bend the knee and slowly return the foot to the floor. Repeat 5 or more times on each side, only lightly touching the floor between each repetition. To increase the difficulty, add a second movement to the sequence: just before the foot is lowered to the floor, straighten the leg and extend it out a few inches above the floor. Then bend the knee once more and return the leg to the starting position. Again, repeat 5 or more times on each side, only lightly touching the floor between each repetition.

b) Next, lie on your back with both legs stretched out on the floor. Place the arms alongside the body, palms facing down. Inhaling, bend one knee and bring it toward the chest. Exhaling, straighten and lengthen the leg, returning it to the floor. Repeat 5 or more times on each side, only lightly touching the floor between each repetition.

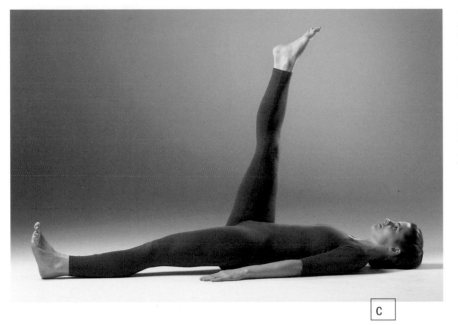

c

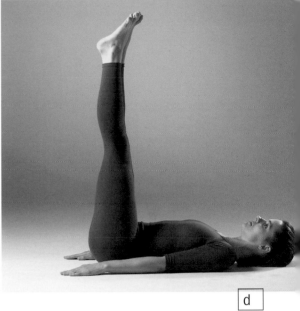

d

c) *Single leglift, straight legs.* Start with both legs extended. Inhaling, press the back of one leg into the floor for support as you raise the other leg. Bend the knee slightly if the hamstrings of the raised leg are tight and restrict the range of movement. Exhaling, lower the leg and alternate sides. Repeat 5 or more times on each side. To increase the level of difficulty raise both legs to 90 degrees. Then lower one leg to just a few inches off the floor and lift it back to 90 degrees. Again, alternate legs, repeating 5 or more times on each side.

d) *Double leglifts.* Lie on your back, knees raised and feet on the floor near the pelvis. Inhaling, lift both knees, then straighten the legs and extend them toward the ceiling. Exhaling, bend the knees and bring the feet back to the floor. Repeat 5 or more times, only lightly touching the floor before lifting again. After a period of practice, increase the level of difficulty: just before the feet reach the floor, straighten the legs and extend them out a few inches above the floor; then bend the knees once more and return the legs to the starting position. Again, repeat 5 or more times, only lightly touching the floor between repetitions.

Next, lie on your back with both legs on the floor. In this variation keep the legs straight as you raise them with an exhalation and lower them with an inhalation. Press the lower back firmly into the floor to prevent strain. Moving continuously—without resting the legs on the floor—is more difficult than releasing the legs to the floor each time. Raise and lower the legs slowly and smoothly with the breath, and keep them straight and aligned as if standing in the mountain pose (p.23). Repeat 5 or more times. Notice if you tend to lead with one side. Often one side is stronger than the other, and does more than its share of work—a good reason to continue with single leglifts along with double leglifts.

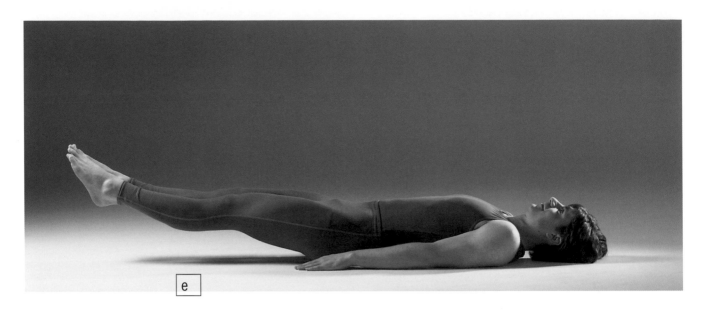

e

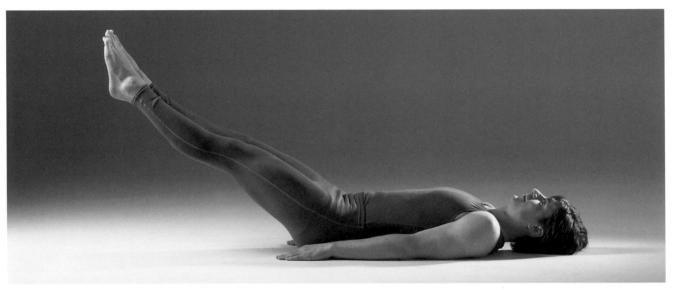

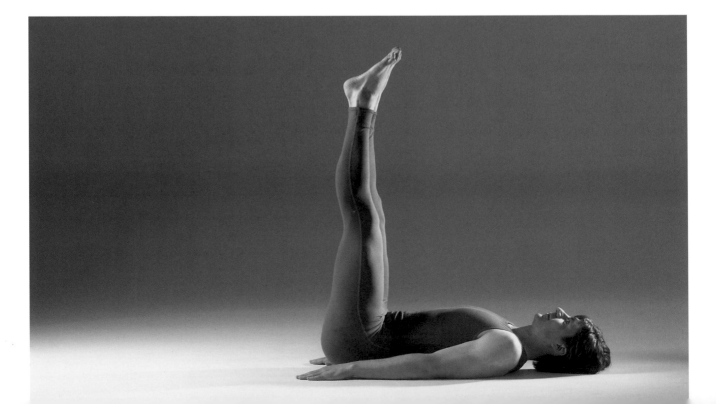

e) *Advanced double leglifts.*

(1) Exhaling, raise both legs about 20 degrees off the floor and hold for 5–20 seconds. (Hold the legs, not the breath!) (2) Next, raise the legs to about 45 degrees and hold again. (3) Finally, raise the legs to 90 degrees and hold once more. Then inhaling, lower back to 45 degrees, then 20 degrees, again holding in each position. Repeat 5 times, resting as necessary between repetitions.

f) *Leglifts and Twist (Jathara Parivartanasana).* Lift the legs to 90 degrees. The arms are on the floor, either perpendicular to the body or overhead. Keeping the knees and ankles together and the upper torso flat on the floor, exhale and lower the straight legs to one side, reaching toward the shoulders with the feet. Hold and breathe, but don't rest the legs on the floor. Then inhale and lift back to center. Repeat on the opposite side. You can also do this as a smooth repetition without holding in any position. Move without strain.

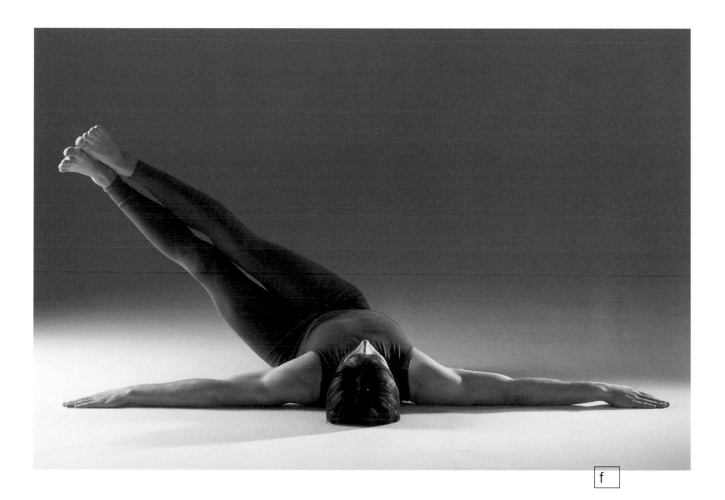

f

Hip-Balance Variations

These poses are intensely energizing. They look deceptively simple, but in the beginning you may be able to stay in the poses for only 1 or 2 breaths.

a) Lie on your back with the knees raised and feet on the floor near the pelvis. The arms are alongside the body with the palms facing in. Press the lower back into the floor and roll the head and upper torso up, looking at your navel center. Now exhale and straighten the left leg, holding it a few inches above the floor. Keep the lower back pressed tightly against the floor as you hold the pose. If you feel strain in the lower back, release the leg and return it to the bent-leg position. After holding on the left side, change and repeat on the right. Over many sessions, gradually work up to a minute on each side.

b) To increase the difficulty of the pose, straighten one leg on the floor and lift the other leg a few inches off the floor.

c) Finally, lift both legs a few inches off the floor. Continue to keep the head lifted and the lower back pressed strongly into the floor. Soften the shoulders, throat, jaw, and face. Keep the navel pressed toward the spine and the lower abdomen firm. You should not be able to slip your hand between the floor and your lower back.

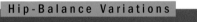

Hip-Balance Variations

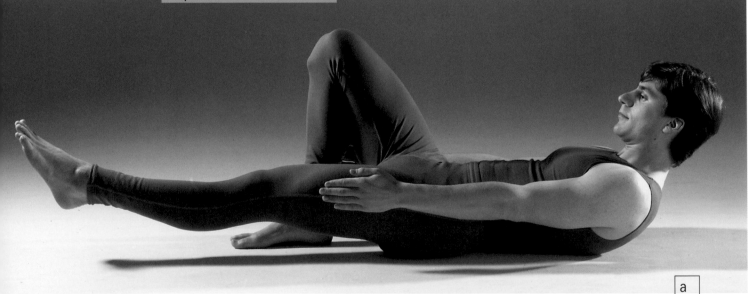

a

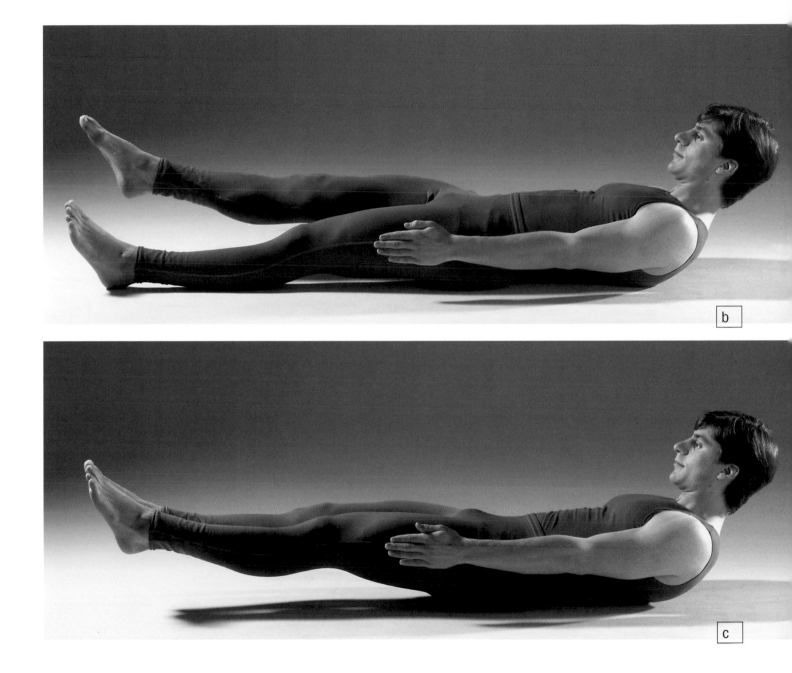

b

c

Plow to Forward Bend

This is a sequence for relatively strong backs. It combines leglifts with abdominal curls, and hence strengthens all the abdominal muscles.

a) To begin, lie on your back with both legs straight out on the floor. The arms may be alongside the body or on the floor above the head.

b) Exhaling, lift both legs, raising the lower back off the floor as the feet move up and overhead. Elevate the pelvis and lift the spine as you bring the feet toward the floor above the head (either parallel to the floor or with the feet touching the floor—the plow pose). Maintain complete control of the movement and do not throw the legs over the head.

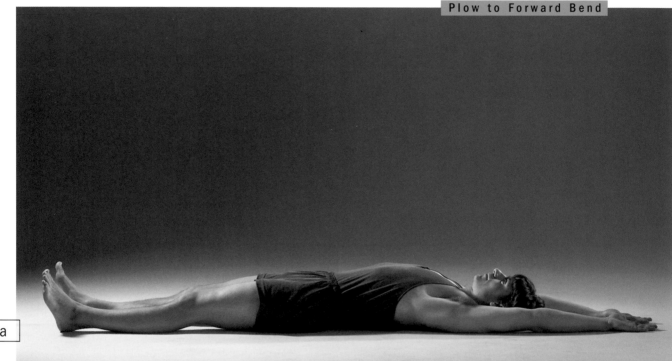

a

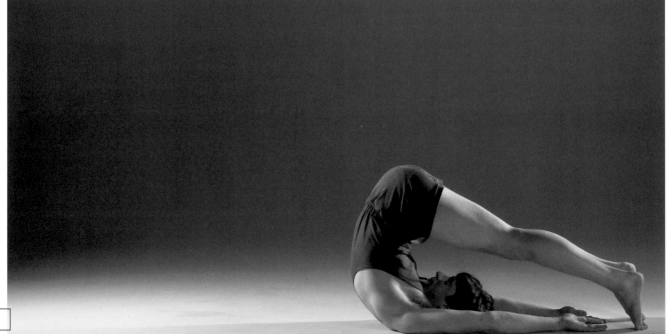

b

c) Next, inhale and slowly uncurl the spine until the pelvis reaches the floor and the legs are again at 90 degrees.

Gripping the floor with the lower back, continue inhaling and lower the legs to the floor.

d) Exhaling, raise the arms, lift the head, and roll to a sitting position, reaching out over the thighs into a forward bend.

Finally, inhaling, round the lower back, and release the spine back to the floor one vertebra at a time until you are again lying flat. Repeat the whole sequence 5 times or more.

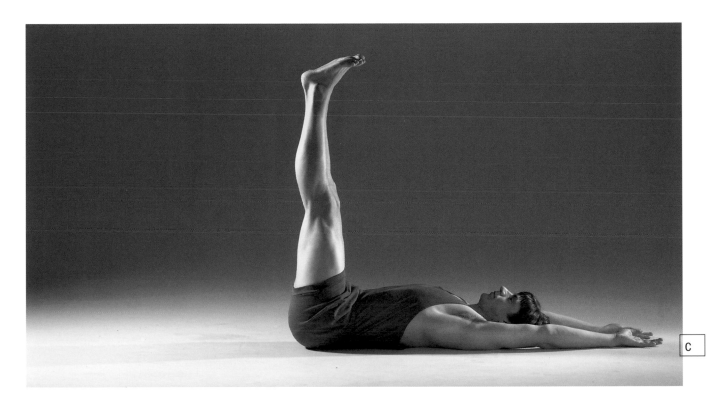

c

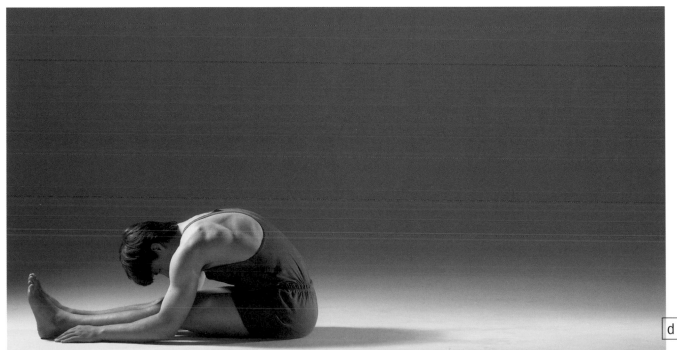

d

Muscles of the Upper Torso—Front View

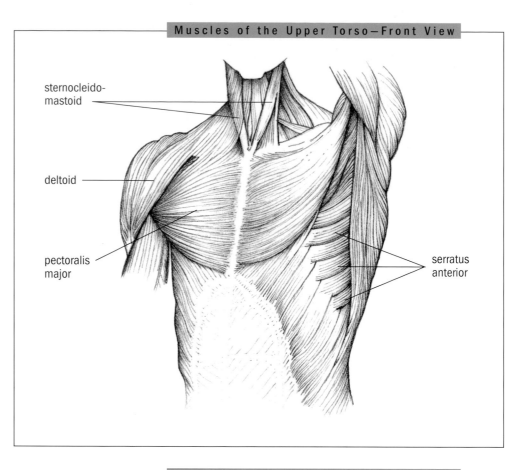

sternocleido-
mastoid

deltoid

pectoralis
major

serratus
anterior

Muscles of the Upper Torso—Rear View

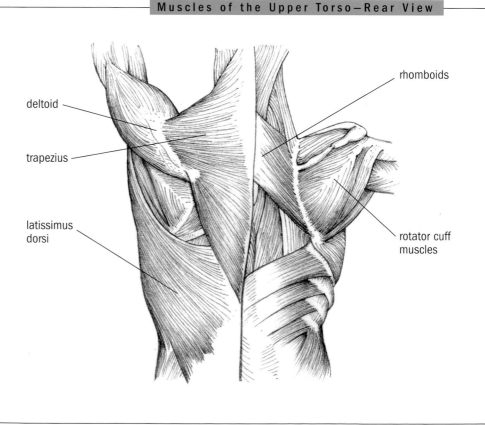

deltoid

trapezius

latissimus
dorsi

rhomboids

rotator cuff
muscles

Shoulders, Arms, and Upper Body

The shoulder joints are among the most mobile in the body, and they permit extensive movements of the arms in all directions. For stability the arms and shoulder joints depend on a stable shoulder girdle (defined as a combination of the two shoulder blades behind, plus the two collarbones and the breastbone in front). This girdle of bone is not complete behind, however, since the two shoulder blades are not interlocked with one another but instead float freely on the back. Some muscles (such as the trapezius) stabilize the shoulder girdle and hold it in place, others (such as the rotator cuff muscles) act on the arms, and yet others (the famous "pecs" and "lats") act directly from the torso to the arms.

Because this region is so complex and yet so mobile, many of these upper body muscles are subject to injury, stiffness, weakness, fatigue, and imbalances of various kinds. Repetitive job- or sports-related stress, emotional tension, movements that habitually misalign the spine, hunching of the shoulders and upper back, and old injuries all contribute to loss of mobility in the shoulders and neck, as well as to pain in the upper back, neck, and head.

To hold all these problems at bay, develop the habit of keeping the shoulders relaxed in daily life. It also helps to keep the head gently lifted, the shoulders down away from the ears, and the movements of the upper body free and easy. The stretches and postures in this section will help you regain proper use and range of movement. To prepare yourself to practice them, concentrate on:

Shoulder rolls p.23

Chest expander p.25

Cat pose twist p.35

Cobra pose pp.36, 94

Cow's face pose, arms p.105

Arch pose p.118

Standing poses Chapters 3 & 5

Sun salutation p.70

Additional Work for Stiff Shoulders and Upper Body

Wall Press

These are excellent tension-relieving shoulder and upper back stretches that can be done anywhere at any time. The secret is to relax and at the same time reach out through the arms.

a) Stand facing a wall, about an arm's length away. Place both hands on the wall at shoulder height, then step back until your feet are parallel and about 3 feet from the wall. Flatten the lower back and bend forward from the hips, keeping the legs straight. The pelvis moves away from the wall, and the head, shoulders, and chest release toward the floor. Press the palms into the wall, and lengthen the inner edges of the arms. Expand the chest, open the armpits, and broaden the upper back. As you hold the stretch, lift the sitting bones and flatten the lower back. Hold and breathe, broadening and lengthening the torso as you inhale, and relaxing tension as you exhale.

b) Next, standing an arm's length from the wall, turn to the left side. Raise the right arm and place the hand on the wall at shoulder height, fingers pointing up. Stand erect with your weight evenly distributed, and keep both shoulders level and relaxed. Press the heel of the hand into the wall, stretching through the length of the arm. Center yourself, breathing smoothly and softening muscles of the face and neck. Intensify the stretch by turning the feet and torso to the left, toward the center of the room. Keep the right hand pressed into the wall and continue to lengthen through the arm. Again, center yourself in the stretch and breathe, relaxing resistance. Then slowly release and repeat on the other side.

Wall Press

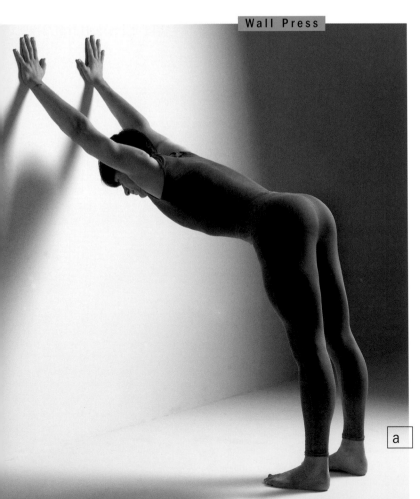

a

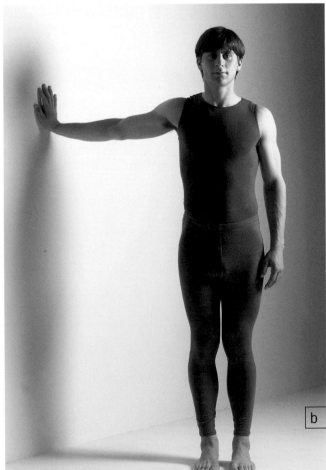

b

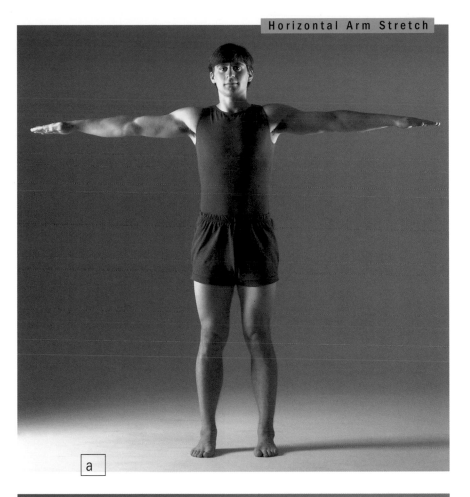

a

Horizontal Arm Stretch

This is a simple pose that is surprisingly energizing.

a) Stand in the mountain pose with the feet parallel and hip-width apart. Inhale and open from the center of the chest, raising the arms to the sides at shoulder height. Lengthen the arms through the fingertips, keeping the shoulder blades drawn down and the tops of the shoulders relaxed. Elongate through the crown of the head, slightly raising the chest. Inhaling, breathe into the sides of the rib cage and abdomen, expanding out through the arms; exhaling, feel the contraction of the torso while maintaining the horizontal stretch in the arms.

b) Bring the feet together. Bend the knees, lowering the pelvis toward the floor and elongating upward through the spine. The arms remain extended from the shoulders. Bend the wrists and press the heels of the hands away from the body as if pressing the hands against a wall. Hold and breathe, lengthening through the arms, feeling the vertical energy of the pose along the axis of the spine and the horizontal energy of the pose along the axis of the arms. When you are ready to release, exhale and lower the arms as you straighten the legs.

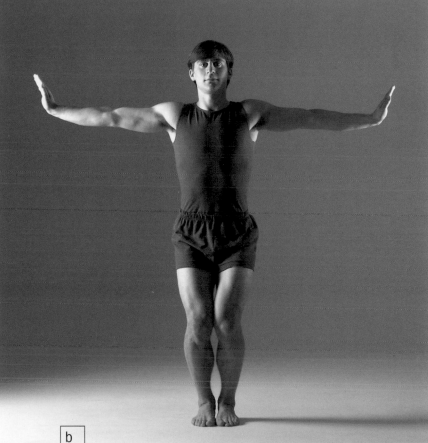

b

Eagle Stretch

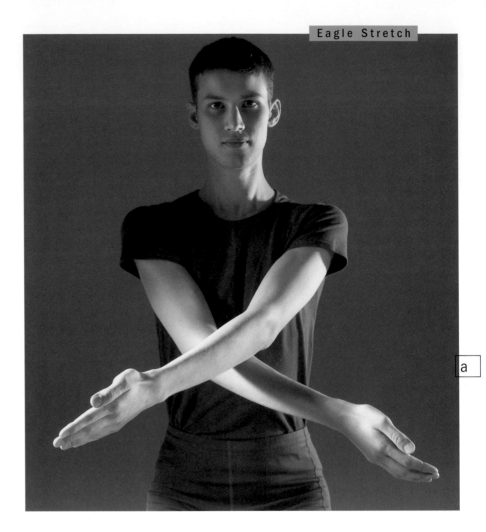

a

Eagle Stretch

This pose stretches that hard-to-reach place between the shoulder blades as well as refreshes the arms.

a) Stand (or sit on a chair) with the spine straight. Smoothly swing your arms across each other at chest height, catching the upper arm just above the elbow joint of the lower arm. Keep the shoulder blades moving down and feel the upper back broadening.

b) Bend the elbows and wrap the forearms so that the palms press together (although they are at different heights). Squeeze the palms and arms together. To intensify the pose, raise the intertwined arms, moving the elbows up and away from the chest. Hold and breathe, relaxing resistance. Release and repeat with the opposite arm on top.

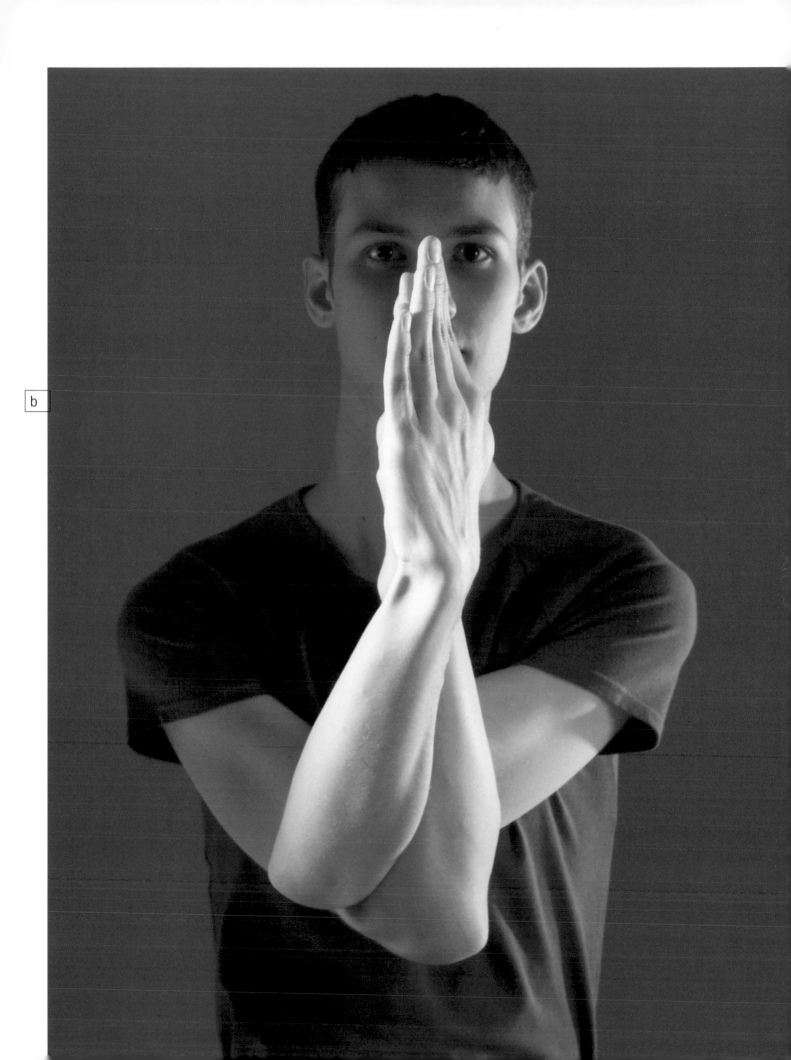

b

Dolphin Pose

The dolphin is one of the best postures for developing strength and flexibility in the shoulders and improving alignment of the upper back and shoulder girdle. It is also an excellent preparation for inverted balance postures like the headstand and forearm balance.

a) Start on your hands and knees, with the knees under the hips and the hands under the shoulders. Lower the forearms to the floor so that the elbows are under the shoulders and the forearms are parallel. Spread the fingers and press the palms and arms into the floor. Now straighten the legs and lift the pelvis, releasing the heels toward the floor and elevating the sitting bones (it's fine, however, if the heels don't touch the floor). Bend the knees slightly if necessary to keep the sitting bones lifting and the chest and shoulders opening. Continue pressing into the forearms, and don't let the elbows spread apart. Broaden the shoulders, pull the shoulder blades down, and open the armpits. Hold and breathe, centering in the pose.

b) For more of a challenge, try the swimming dolphin. Exhale and shift your weight forward. The chest moves toward the floor between the forearms, and the face to the hands or beyond. Then inhale and press down through the forearms, shifting your weight back, moving the chest behind the arms toward the thighs, head in line with the elbows. Try to press the chest further behind the arms than you have experienced in the static stationary dolphin position. Repeat 5–10 times (this is hard!), breathing deeply and coordinating the movement with the breath. Then rest in the child's pose.

176

Dolphin Pose

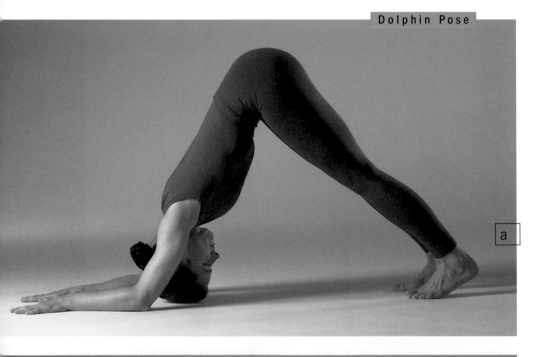

a

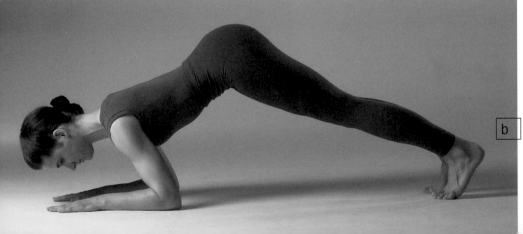

b

Eight-Point Pose
(Ashtanamaskara)

This pose uses the position and weight of the body on the floor to focus a gentle backward bend in the upper back, where it's most difficult to open the back. It also stretches the front of the neck and throat. You may want to follow this posture with the crocodile pose (p.20).

a) Start on your hands and knees, with the knees under the hips and the hands under the shoulders. Arch the spine, bend the elbows, and lower the chest and chin to the floor between the hands. Move the knees back or further apart as necessary to allow the chest to rest on the floor. Stretch the front of the neck so that the face looks forward, the chin is on the floor, and the throat is pressed toward the floor. Pull the shoulder blades down and together. Breathe deeply and relax. If the pose creates strain, take some of the weight onto the hands (which are still under the shoulders or alongside the chest), and soften the chest and throat.

b) To further deepen the pose, move the knees toward the chest, and stretch the arms out on the floor, perpendicular to the body.

c) In the most advanced arm position, bring the palms together behind the back (the reverse prayer pose) and wiggle the hands up the spine, letting the fingers reach for the back of the head. Since this version of the pose offers no arm support, practice it only after you are comfortable with the two supported versions.

Eight-Point Pose

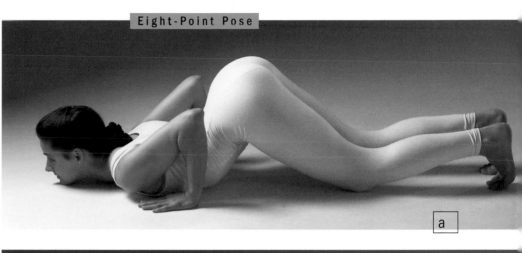

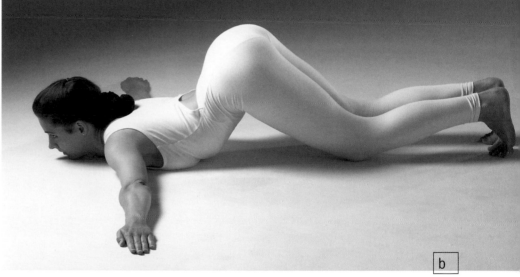

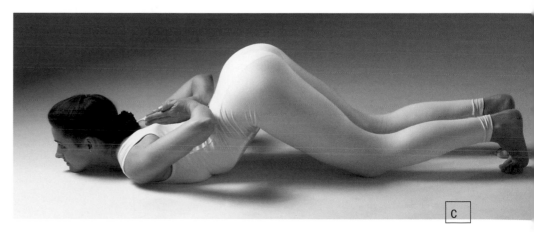

All-Fours Cat Twist

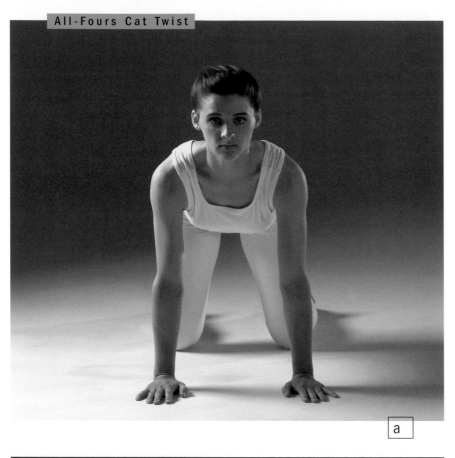

a

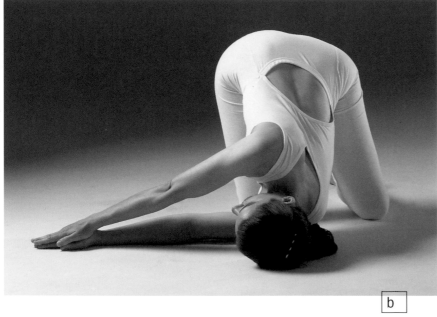

b

All-Fours Cat Twist

This powerful twist opens the hips, spine, and shoulders. It is an especially effective stretch for the intercostal muscles (the muscles between the ribs).

a) Start on your hands and knees.

b) Slide the left arm under the right shoulder and place the back of the left shoulder on the floor. The left arm extends out along the floor and the head is turned enough to stretch the back of the neck away from the shoulder. Place the palm of the right hand on the left palm. Adjust the position of the knees by moving one or both knees further from the chest or further apart to stabilize the pose and elongate the spine.

c) Lift the right arm to open the chest, reaching straight up first, then bending the elbow and placing the hand at the back of the waist. Breathe and expand the chest, moving the right shoulder and ribs back, and the left shoulder and ribs forward.

d) Stretch the right arm up and then back toward the floor behind you, keeping the shoulder pulled down away from the ear. Stretch the back of the right shoulder and upper back toward the floor, rolling the face toward the ceiling. Feel the chest expand on the inhalation. With each exhalation deepen the twist, allowing gravity to draw the right arm down, gently opening the spine, ribs, and shoulder. Slowly reverse to come out of the twist. Arch the spine in the cat pose (p.32) a few times to release any tension. Then repeat on the other side, again finishing with a few repetitions of the cat pose.

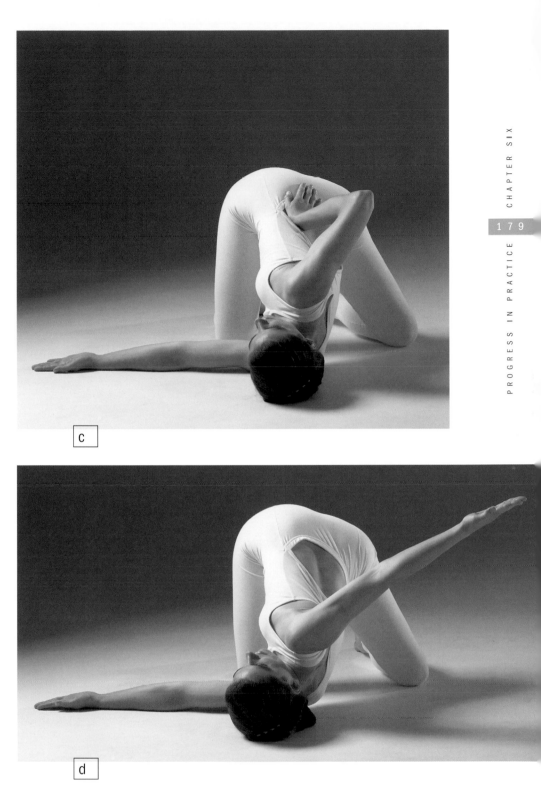

c

d

Upward-Facing Plank Pose (Purvottanasana)

The plank pose opens the chest, strengthens and opens the shoulders, and generally tones the muscles of the back of the body.

a) Start by sitting in the staff pose (p.102) with the legs straight out in front of you. Place the hands flat on the floor and a little behind the hips with the fingers pointed forward. Press the tailbone down and elongate the spine through the crown of the head. Keep the legs active by lifting the kneecaps and reaching out through the heels. Lift the sternum and draw the shoulder blades down.

b) Exhaling, lift the pelvis and the chest toward the ceiling, supporting yourself on your hands and pressing the soles of the feet toward the floor. Point the toes and lengthen through the balls of the feet as you lift the chest. Stretch the head back to open the front of the neck, but lengthen the neck at the same time to avoid compressing the vertebrae there. Deepen the pose for several breaths. Then lower the pelvis and return to the staff pose. Repeat several times to build strength.

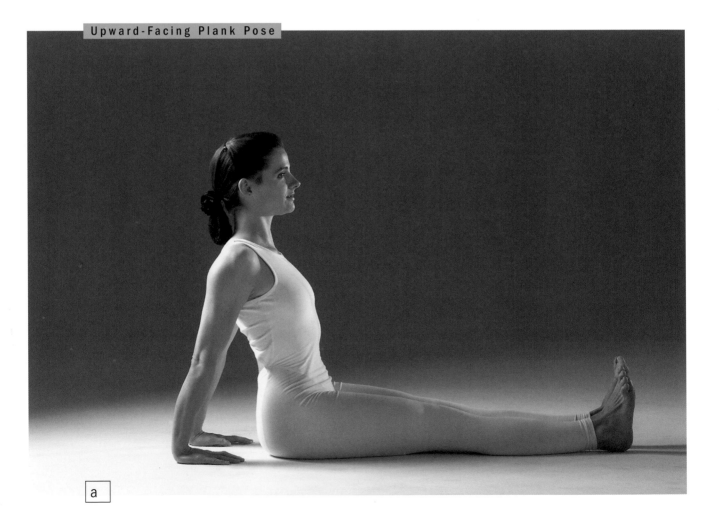

Upward-Facing Plank Pose

a

This chapter has explored ways to expand the practice of yoga asanas and to work with common problem areas. The inner ease which comes from regular practice will naturally give you confidence, and it will not take long to begin creating practice routines tailored to meet the needs of your day. At the same time, you may be ready to explore a new aspect of yoga to add to your practice: the more subtle breathing techniques for which yoga is well-known. If so, you are ready for the next chapter: pranayama.

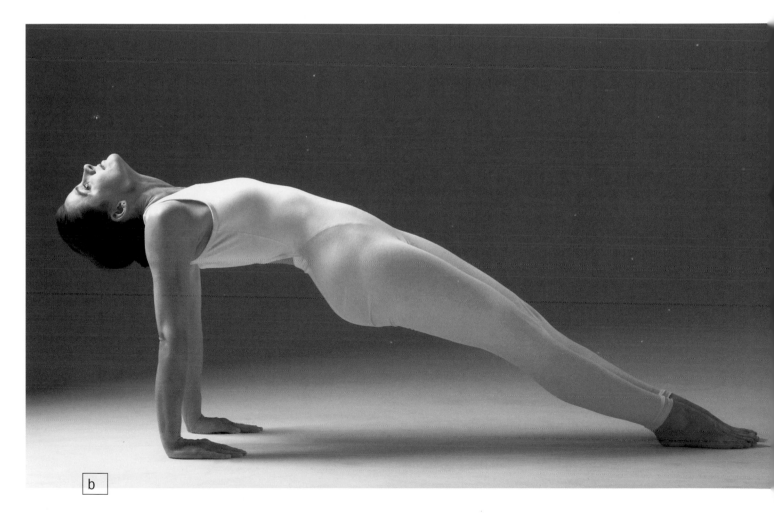

b

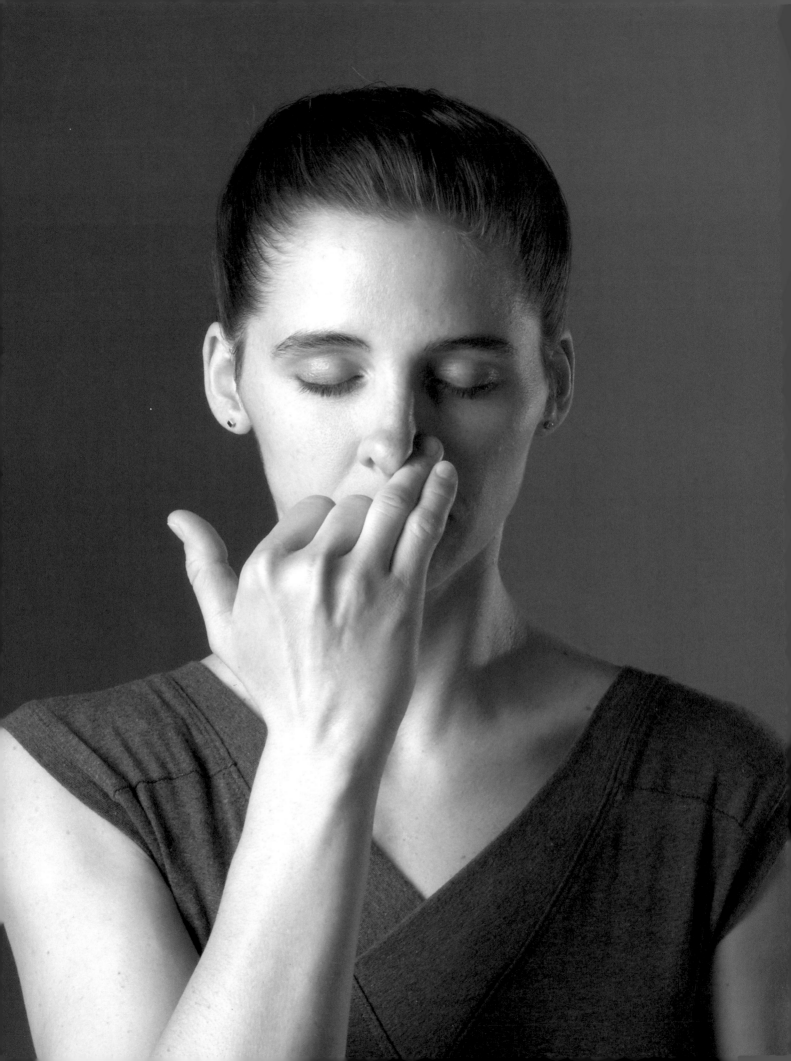

CHAPTER SEVEN

PRANAYAMA

By the regular and systematic practice
of pranayama I have gained a state of purity,
and I am not disturbed even when the
axis of the Earth is shaken.

—— *Yoga Vasishtha*

T H E   yogis tell us that the mind and the body are interconnected by a complex and vibrant system of inner energy which is sustained by the ebb and flow of the breath. Thus energy, breath, and life are inextricably linked. Practices that make us conscious of this system constitute a science called *pranayama*, a vast and intriguing branch of yoga in which one's innate vital energy is brought to awareness, gradually regulated, and integrated into the practice of concentration. Pranayama is the fourth rung in the classic raja yoga system.

The word *pranayama* is a compound of two words: *prana*, meaning "life force" or "vital energy," and *yama*, meaning "to regulate" or "to control." Pranayama is the

yogic science of balancing and regulating vital energy through the skillful manipulation of breath. The word is also used by yoga adepts to mean that these techniques expand our energy and ultimately lead to vibrant health and the realization of spiritual goals.

The practice of pranayama varies somewhat from school to school, but every tradition recommends a systematic approach. The first stage in the process—mastering relaxed, diaphragmatic breathing—has been described in chapter 4. You may need to review the practices outlined there if you are uncertain about them.

Advanced pranayama exercises, including any that involve breath retention, must be learned under the direct supervision of a qualified teacher who can model the practices and provide experienced guidance. But even though a book cannot take the place of a teacher, the following exercises have been carefully prepared with the beginning student in mind: the instructions are intended to provide a safe and effective practice of introductory-level techniques. If you are uncertain about any aspect of a particular technique, simply discontinue practicing until you can obtain personal guidance.

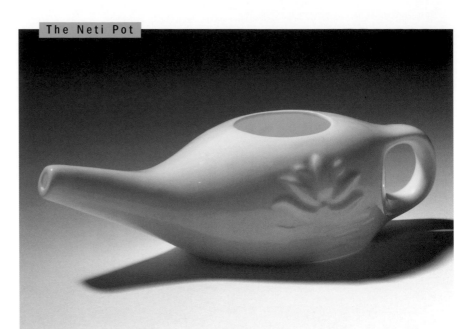

The Neti Pot

Five practices are described: the nasal wash, the complete breath, *agni sara, kapalabhati,* and *nadi shodhanam.* They can be integrated into your daily yoga schedule as the need and interest arise. But remember that your practice is meant to serve you, not the other way around. Let a balance of self-discipline and common sense guide you as you develop your routine.

The Nasal Wash

The purpose of the nasal wash is exactly what the name suggests: to cleanse the nasal passageways and maintain healthy tissue functioning. Remember from chapter 4 that within the nose are cells that secrete mucus (which lubricates the nose and provides a protective lining for the airways that extend down to the throat).

The mucus lining also traps dust as well as potentially infectious microbes such as bacteria, viruses, and fungi. Antibodies in the mucus help protect the body from these invaders (in a healthy person mucus carries microbes from the nose into the stomach, through the bowels, and eventually transports them out of the body). So long as it is of a healthy consistency, the mucus blanket is carried along by the underlying cilia and is completely replaced every 10–20 minutes. However, when the blanket becomes thin and watery, mucus pools, running out the

nose and back into the throat (postnasal drip). Thick or excessive mucus, on the other hand, overwhelms the cilia, leading to congestion which may clog sinus openings and prevent the sinuses from draining.

Practices for cleansing the nose and improving the health of the nasal lining have been described since ancient times. One of the best involves what is called a *neti pot,* a small spouted vessel used to pass a saline solution from one nostril to the other. Far from being uncomfortable, in a short time this simple procedure can become one of your most satisfying practices.

THE TECHNIQUE

Fill the neti pot with a warm (body temperature) saline solution. It is best to use a pure, non-iodized salt, such as kosher salt or canning/pickling salt—the amount depends on how finely the salt is ground. Use a slightly rounded half-teaspoonful with coarse varieties, like kosher salt, and a heaping quarter-teaspoonful with finely ground salt, such as non-iodized table salt. Make sure the salt is completely dissolved. If you have just the right amount (not too much and not too little), the solution won't burn; in fact it is soothing. As it passes through the nose it picks up excess mucus and carries it out. And if there is an inflammation in the nose, the salt in the solution draws out fluid from swollen tissues.

The technique can be mastered in a few tries.

▶ Begin by leaning over the sink, face downward.

▶ Twist your head to the side, which will raise one nostril.

▶ Breathe through the mouth (holding the breath is not necessary and may even prevent the water from flowing smoothly).

▶ Insert the spout into the upper nostril and let the water flow through the nose and out the lower nostril.

▶ Empty the pot into one nostril, then refill it and do the same thing with the other nostril. Or you may use half a potful on each side. Either way, be sure to do the practice on both sides of the nose.

The head position is important. If water flows into your mouth instead of out the lower nostril, you are too erect and the water is flowing into your throat: lower your head a little. If the water does not flow into the other nostril you may need to either raise your head or twist further. Success comes easily with a little experi-

mentation. If the flow won't start, consult a qualified teacher. Normally the problem is simple to correct.

Once the nasal wash has been completed, 5–10 moderately forceful exhalations will help clear the nose of any loose mucus and remaining water. It is important, however, not to squeeze the nose or block the nostrils during these exhalations, and to keep the mouth at least partially open (otherwise water or mucus can be propelled back into the openings of the Eustachian tubes). Blow firmly out into the sink, or into a tissue held lightly around the nose. Remember that one purpose of the wash is to reduce excess mucus—so don't be squeamish about blowing it out. You'll feel better if you do.

If there is still some saline solution in the nose, selected yoga postures are sometimes used to help clear it because they tilt the head in one direction or another to assist draining. Two yoga poses commonly recommended are a simple forward bend and a rotated forward bend with the head turned upward. You can experiment to find the position(s) most useful to you. When you come out of the posture, liquid may trickle from the nose. Blow it out gently, and follow with another round of moderately forceful exhalations.

Head Position in the Nasal Wash

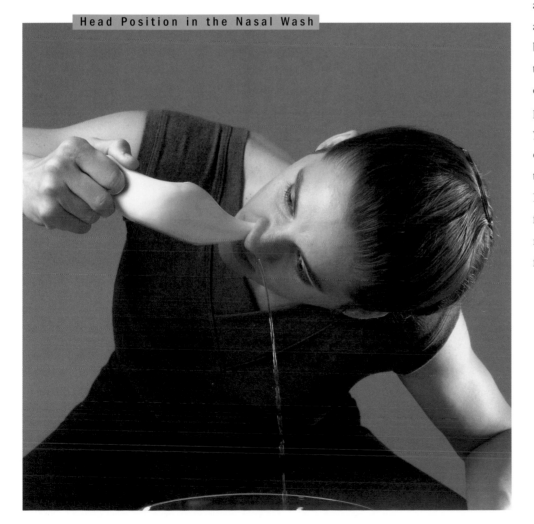

Simple Forward Bend

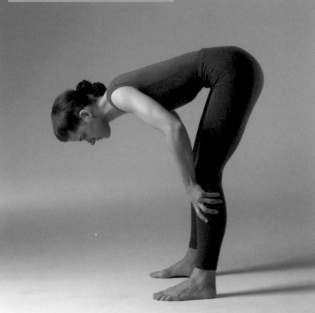

Twisting Bend

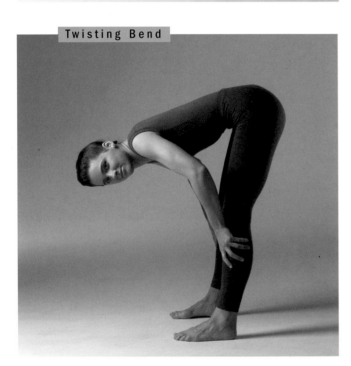

▶ <u>Benefits and Cautions</u>: The nasal wash is beneficial for anyone and can be practiced even by those who do not have any other familiarity with yoga. An obvious benefit of the nasal wash is that it rinses away excess mucus. But it is not intended simply for those with nasal congestion. If you are looking for other reasons to try it, here's a baker's dozen.

▶ Your nose will feel clean even after you have been breathing in a dusty or sooty environment.

▶ Your breath will flow more easily and quietly. This is relaxing at a deep level.

▶ With regular practice, your sense of smell will improve.

▶ As smell improves, the sense of taste improves.

▶ Blockage at the opening of the Eustachian tubes can be relieved.

▶ Openings from the sinus canals into the nose may drain more easily, preventing or relieving a variety of sinus-related conditions (the saline solution, however, does not enter the sinuses).

▶ According to yoga manuals, the optic nerve is soothed by the nearby flow of water, relaxing the eyes.

▶ With regular practice chronic inflammation and irritability of the mucus lining in the nose can be improved. Normal, healthy nasal function can be restored.

▶ The anxiety or discomfort created by nasal congestion is relieved.

▶ Dependence on over-the-counter nasal sprays and drops can be reduced or eliminated.

▶ Symptoms of hayfever, dust, and other airborne allergies can be relieved.

▶ Yoga breathing practices and concentration of attention are made easier.

▶ Unnecessary mouth breathing can be reduced or eliminated.

One word of caution: the nasal wash is not a substitute for medical attention, and anyone with chronic inflammation or blockage of the nasal passages should seek expert assistance.

SOME FINAL THOUGHTS

Once you have purchased a neti pot, plan to use it daily for 3–6 days as you learn to do the wash. Then experiment to find how often you need to do it and the time of day most suitable for you. Here are some suggestions.

► Try using the neti pot every morning for one month to see its overall effects.

► Do the nasal wash before your asana or meditation practice.

► Rinse your nose promptly after exposure to dusty, smoky, or sooty environments and notice the relief.

► Anticipate allergy seasons by getting started on a regular schedule of two or more daily rinsings.

► In general, use the neti pot before meals, rather than following meals, to harmonize with the body's natural mucus-producing schedule.

A person who regularly drinks water through the nose in the early morning at the end of the night becomes intelligent, develops eyesight as acute as an eagle, is spared the graying of hair and the wrinkling of skin, and is freed from all diseases.

—from the Yoga-Ratnakara, *a treatise on Ayurvedic medicine*

The Complete Breath

Considering that the average lung capacity is 4,000–5,000 ml, the amount of air exchanged in normal breathing is surprisingly small. Everyday breathing transports only about 500 ml of air, or 10 percent of the lung capacity, in and out of the body, but this seemingly meager amount is more than adequate. If breathing is relatively continuous, it supplies all the body's needs.

During periods of fatigue, however, or as a break from the rapid pace of the day, you can get a refreshing pick-me-up by breathing more deeply for a few breaths. This practice, called the complete breath, is not meant to replace normal breathing, but you may find, with a little practice, that it becomes a regular feature of your day.

The complete breath employs three styles of breathing: diaphragmatic, thoracic, and clavicular. When they are merged systematically in the complete breath, they expand the lungs to near-maximum capacity.

► Diaphragmatic breathing draws air into the lowest portion of the lungs and supplies the best exchange of blood gases. And since the practice is done in the corpse pose, diaphragmatic breathing will expand the abdomen, while the rib cage remains still.

► Thoracic breathing expands the chest and the middle portion of the lungs. Movements here are the result of the intercostal muscles which lie between the ribs.

► Clavicular breathing (at the level of the collar bones) uses the muscles of the neck and shoulders to fill the uppermost part of the lungs.

With practice you will soon be able to distinguish among the three styles of breathing and use them to expand the lungs.

THE TECHNIQUE

- ▶ Lie in the corpse pose and establish smooth, diaphragmatic breathing. Let your abdomen rise and fall with each breath—eliminating pauses, jerks, and unnecessary sounds.

- ▶ Begin the complete breath by inhaling diaphragmatically, filling the lower portion of the lungs and fully expanding the abdomen.

- ▶ When the diaphragm cannot be contracted further, continue inhaling by expanding the chest. Breathe at the same pace throughout the exercise.

- ▶ Finally, when the chest is fully expanded, shift to the muscles in the uppermost part of the torso and neck—without straining or creating exaggerated tension.

- ▶ When this last effort is complete you have inhaled to your full inspiratory capacity and are ready to exhale at the same pace as the inhalation.

- ▶ Exhale in reverse order: slowly release the breath by relaxing the contraction of the neck and shoulder muscles; the intercostal muscles; and finally the diaphragm.

- ▶ Repeat for a total of 5 breaths. Then resume normal diaphragmatic breathing and come back to a sitting posture.

HINTS AND CAUTIONS

Because the complete breath relieves fatigue and is generally energizing, you will find it effective at the end of a workday or at any other time of unusually low energy. Do not strain at any point in the exercise. Let the inhalation and exhalation flow smoothly at a pace that is natural and unhurried, one that can be sustained over the length of all 5 breaths.

Agni Sara

One of the most common signs of physical decline is the loss of muscle tone in the abdominal wall. To reverse this process we must rebuild muscle strength and rekindle abdominal fire. Among the practices that accomplish this, *agni sara* ("energizing the abdominal fire") is particularly effective.

The navel area is the fireplace, the furnace, of the physical body. Before birth the body receives nourishment and life through the umbilical cord, and after birth this area functions as the center of digestive fire. At a more subtle level this is the region through which life-sustaining energy circulates. In addition to the digestive system, the fire at the navel center energizes and empowers the other systems of the body, including the eliminative and immune systems, and thus it has a positive effect on the body's ability to cleanse and heal itself.

The navel center is the genesis of good physical health as well as success in both worldly pursuits and spiritual unfoldment. The fire here helps us gather strength to begin the process of self-transformation. Like a miniature star, the navel center is a hub of power and light; it is the solar plexus, the sun-like center of energy.

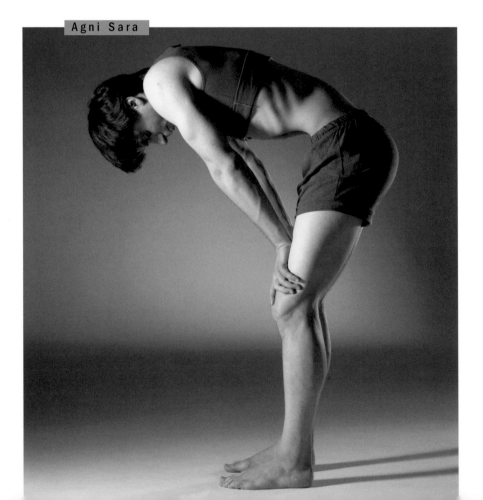

Agni Sara

FIRST STAGE OF PRACTICE

Agni sara is most easily learned in two stages. The first, called *akunchana prasarana* (the abdominal squeeze), is pictured and described as part of Asana Sequence One (p.30). For convenience, here are the instructions:

Stand with the feet slightly wider than hip-width apart. Bend your knees and lean forward, placing the hands on the thighs. Settle the weight of the torso on the arms, relaxing the abdomen. Exhale and firmly contract the abdominal muscles, pressing the navel toward the spine. Then, as you inhale, relax and let the abdomen return to its normal position. Repeat 10 times.

This movement massages the internal organs. It alternately compresses the abdomen as you exhale (which squeezes blood out of the abdominal cavity) and relaxes the abdomen as you inhale (which enriches the organs with a fresh supply of oxygen-rich blood). This cleansing and nourishing action affects all the organs and results in improved digestion, improved elimination, increased assimilation of nutrients, and increased circulation. The abdominal squeeze also improves circulation of the lymph in this region, thus eliminating wastes. It provides mild stimulation to the cardiovascular system and gently massages the heart and lungs. The abdominal contractions increase the strength of the abdominal muscles, which are essential for proper posture and breathing. And as strength and awareness of these muscles improves, the decline of abdominal health is prevented and even reversed.

SECOND STAGE OF PRACTICE

In the second stage of practice, agni sara proper, control of the abdominal movement is further refined as muscles deep in the base of the abdomen are brought to awareness. As before, movements are coordinated with the breath.

▶ Stand with the feet slightly wider than hip-width apart. Bend your knees and lean forward, placing the hands on the thighs. Settle the weight of the torso on the arms with elbows straight.

▶ Exhaling, slowly contract the muscles just above the pubic bone at the very base of the abdomen, pressing firmly inward and upward. This contraction will also create strong upward pressure in the perineum (the area between the genitals and the anus). Continue exhaling, and move the contraction of the abdominal wall upward toward the rib cage.

▶ At the end of the exhalation inhale and slowly release the contraction from the upper abdomen back down to the base. The motion will feel wave-like as it moves from the base upward, and from the upper abdomen downward. There is no pause in the movement of the breath or abdomen.

▶ Contractions are firm, but not strained. There is no sense of air hunger or discomfort when you breathe. Be attentive and listen to your body. Repeat 15 times.

▶ Benefits and Cautions: Agni sara intensifies the benefits of the abdominal squeeze, and it is even recommended for students of advanced age. Agni sara works against the force of gravity, reversing the downward shift in the contents of the abdominal cavity that contributes to a variety of diseases of old age. It improves the functioning of the bowels, bladder, digestive system, nervous system, circulatory system, and reproductive system.

Those with cardiovascular disease or high blood pressure, however, should consult with their physician before beginning either of the practices described here. The practices are not recommended for anyone with a stomach ulcer or hiatal hernia, or for pregnant women. Women should not do these exercises during their menstrual period (agni sara stimulates an upward flow of energy that is counter to the natural cleansing flow at that time). Finally, the stomach must be empty during these practices. Generally, this means waiting three hours following a normal meal.

It is unusual for the muscles of the lower abdomen to be isolated and contracted; hence you may experience stiffness in the beginning. With regular practice, however, the abdominal wall will soon strengthen and the movement will become smooth. Then gradually increase the number of repetitions: 20–30 repetitions in a day is a solid practice that will yield many benefits.

This practice does not need to be done at the same time as other postures, and so the total number of repetitions can be spread throughout the day. The best times are in the early morning, before meals, or in the evening. Occasional practice is never fruitless, but regular repetition results in the greatest gain.

Kapalabhati

Kapalabhati (*kapala* means "skull" and *bhati* means "to shine or to be lustrous") is said to make the skull shine by cleansing the nasal passageways and sinuses and ultimately supplying the brain with fresh, oxygen-rich blood. It also cleanses the throat and lungs and stimulates the abdominal muscles and organs.

Most of the many yoga breathing practices emphasize muscular control during inhalation, not exhalation. Kapalabhati reverses this pattern: here it is the exhalation that is active, and the inhalation passive. And unlike most yoga breathing exercises, kapalabhati is initially energizing rather than calming; cleansing and heating, rather than cooling.

THE TECHNIQUE

Kapalabhati is practiced in a seated pose, and it is important to maintain a steady posture during the practice. Make sure that the head, neck, and trunk are erect and that your body is stable and comfortable.

The essence of kapalabhati is a steady repetition of forceful exhalations followed by slower, passive, inhalations. Each outward breath is propelled by a powerful inward thrust of the abdomen; following this thrust the abdomen is relaxed and the breath automatically flows back into the lungs, recoiling from the force of the exhalation. Each inhalation is smooth and effortless and prepares the respiratory system for the next strike of the abdomen, which again drives air up and out through the nose. A cycle of exhalation and inhalation is counted as one breath, and a prescribed number of repetitions is completed depending on the capacity of the student. All breaths are through the nose.

The correct practice of kapalabhati produces a clear, crisp sound as the breath leaves the nostrils. The air passing through the throat does not interfere with the sound, and the cheeks always remain in place without puffing out. The exhalation in kapalabhati is created by

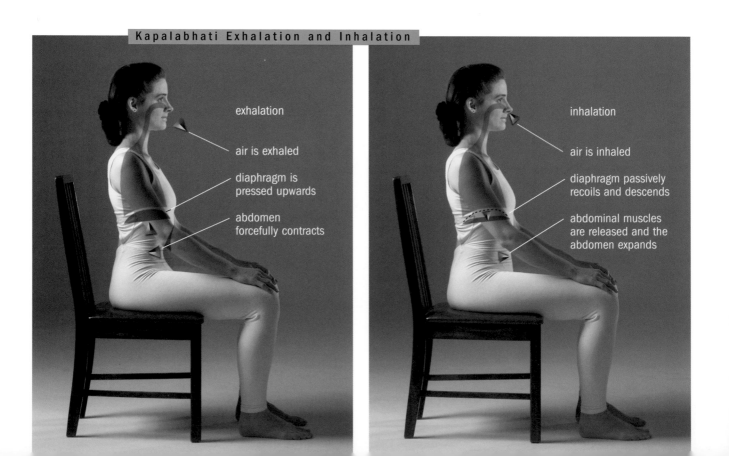

Kapalabhati Exhalation and Inhalation

exhalation

air is exhaled

diaphragm is pressed upwards

abdomen forcefully contracts

inhalation

air is inhaled

diaphragm passively recoils and descends

abdominal muscles are released and the abdomen expands

the inward-thrusting abdomen, not by other accessory muscles, and it is important not to involve the muscles of the chest, the shoulders, or the neck and face in the vigorous contractions.

PICKING UP SPEED

After a little practice, when the movements of the breath seem comfortable, you must establish a rhythmic pace. A good starting rate is about one second for exhalation and 2–3 seconds for inhalation. You may increase the speed gradually; however, it is important not to sacrifice the vigor of the abdominal contractions merely for the sake of going faster. And whatever the speed, the breaths are always nasal and there are no pauses between them.

▶Benefits and Cautions: Kapalabhati is a breathing exercise with connections to many systems of yoga practice. It is one of six practices *(shat kriyas)* taught in hatha yoga for internal cleansing—it purifies the lungs, the air passageways, and the subtle nerve currents, or *nadis*. It is energizing and heating, and because of its effect on the respiratory center, a few rounds are also done before more advanced pranayama practices.

Kapalabhati oxygenates the blood: thus it renews body tissues and helps to arrest the process of aging. It is said to correct ailments arising from coldness, and it is beneficial for nerves, circulation, and metabolism. It is said to invigorate the lungs and increase respiratory capacity. If you are trying to stop smoking, the practice of kapalabhati followed by breath awareness in the crocodile pose will be helpful.

As in all breathing practices, there are cautions to be followed. Kapalabhati is not to be practiced by persons with high or low blood pressure or with coronary heart disease. Those who have problems with their eyes (e.g., glaucoma), ears (e.g., fluid in the ears), or a bleeding nose should not practice this exercise. For these problems consult with a physician who is familiar with the practice.

Always practice on an empty stomach, two or more hours after eating. Stop if you experience pain in your side, if you feel dizzy, or if you are unable to maintain a steady rhythm. Most important, pay full attention to your capacity. This practice will build stamina if it is allowed to develop over time. Whenever signs of fatigue develop, end your practice.

ESTABLISHING A PRACTICE

Practice kapalabhati twice a day. Because these breaths can be energizing it is usually best to do this in the morning and either late afternoon or early evening rather than just before bedtime. In the context of a full yoga practice, kapalabhati comes at the end of your posture routine and before alternate nostril breathing and meditation. This will reduce physical and mental lethargy and keep the mind alert and refreshed.

In order to establish a practice of kapalabhati, keep three objectives in mind:

▶ Build abdominal strength to create forceful contractions.
▶ Gradually increase the speed of the breaths to the desired pace.
▶ Gradually increase the number of repetitions.

The practice is done in rounds. In the beginning 11 expulsions of air constitute one round, and 1–3 rounds are completed at one sitting. Pause between rounds and breathe normally to rest and relax your nervous system. You can slowly increase the number of repetitions in a round, but always stay within your capacity.

Caduceus

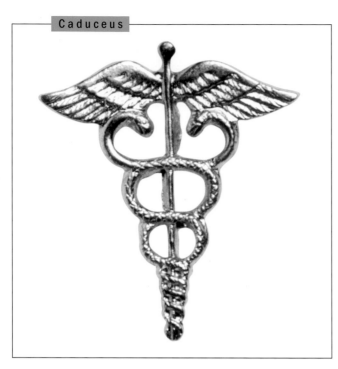

Nadis along the Spine

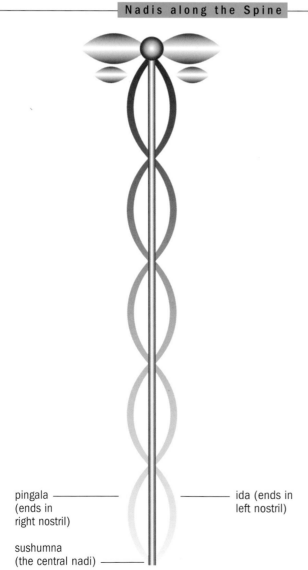

pingala ——————— ida (ends in
(ends in   left nostril)
right nostril)

sushumna
(the central nadi) ———

The pranayama practice called *nadi shodhanam*, or channel purification, is a cleansing exercise that both unblocks and balances the flow of vital energy by alternately passing the breath through one nostril and then the other (giving rise to the other common English name for nadi shodhanam: "alternate nostril breathing"). The practice calms the nervous system and is frequently used just prior to meditation.

In the practice of yoga the nostrils are not merely passive entranceways for air, they are gateways to the vast system of energy within. Nadi shodhanam brings our attention to these gates and slowly develops sensitivity to the sensations that accompany the breath as it flows in each nostril. And once we have developed awareness of these sensations, the flow of breath in the nostrils becomes an internal reference that provides new and helpful information about our inner functioning.

The word *nadi* means "river," or "channel"; the nadis are flowing currents of energy. The system of nadis is composed of many thousands of major channels and related tributaries, branches, and intersections. Among them, three govern our overall functioning and determine the general tone of the entire system. They lie along the spinal column, two twining upward on either side, and one rising directly upward in the center. The channel ending in the left nostril is called *ida; pingala* ends in the right nostril; and *sushumna* rises centrally along the spine to the base of the skull. This configuration can be seen not only in traditional yogic symbolism but also in the art of other ancient cultures. The ancient Greek image of the caduceus, for example, the symbol of medicine, is a case in point.

THE NASAL CYCLE

If you observe the breath in your nostrils at this moment, you will probably find that one nostril is flowing more freely than the other or that one nostril is almost completely blocked while the other carries most of the airstream to and from the lungs. This means that one nostril is active and the other passive. (If you have difficulty determining which nostril is flowing more freely, hold a pocket mirror under your nose and breathe on it: the pattern of moisture formed on the mirror from the open nostril will be larger.)

This difference is the result of a natural alternation in nostril dominance that takes place throughout the day and night—in modern research it is called the "nasal cycle." When the cycle is relatively regular, and the shifting results in a moderate rather than an extreme difference in nostril dominance, the cycle is balanced; when the cycle includes long periods of dominance on one side, or when one nostril seems almost entirely blocked, the cycle is imbalanced. Imbalances in the nasal cycle are associated with changes in mood, with agitation, and with problems in concentrating. When one nostril is entirely blocked it is more difficult to meditate.

There are many ways to bring the nasal cycle into balance. For example, regulating sleep, food, sexual activity, and exercise patterns can help to stabilize the flow of breath. But in the long run the best way is a regular and balanced yoga routine, including nadi shodhanam (which is said to balance both irregularity and extreme swinging in the cycle).

As the nasal cycle returns to balance, nadi shodhanam also works to cleanse and strengthen the system of nadis, and this leads to deeper awareness. The breath becomes slower and more refined, and with experience a natural inwardness develops that is delightful and calming to the mind.

PRELIMINARIES

The techniques for practicing channel purification are quite specific.

▶ Sit erect. The posture of the spine during channel purification is crucial—if the practice is done with a bent spine, it can disrupt the nervous system and increase physical and mental tension. A well-known teacher in India described practicing nadi shodhanam with a rounded back as the equivalent of bombarding the spine with a hydraulic jackhammer!

▶ Breathe diaphragmatically and without pause. In the process of concentrating on manipulating the nostrils it is easy to lose touch with one's own breathing. The breath should remain deep, smooth, relaxed, and diaphragmatic during the entire exercise. Gradually the length of the breath will increase.

▶ Close off the nostrils by lightly pressing the small flap of skin at either side of the nose. This is done with a special hand position, a *mudra,* in which the index and middle fingers of the hand are curled to touch the base of the thumb, opening a space between the thumb and ring finger for the nose. The thumb is used to close one nostril and the ring finger is used to close the other.

▶ And finally, during the practice of channel purification it is common to see students focusing so much on manipulating the nose that they bend the head forward. Or they may be applying too much pressure on the nostrils with the finger and thumb, thus bending the nose to the side. Remember that the nose should not be distorted during the practice nor the balanced alignment of the head and neck altered. Close the nostrils lightly.

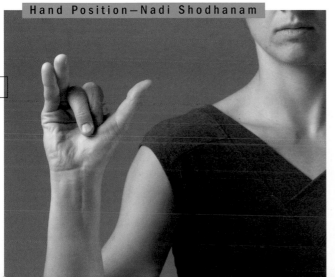

Hand Position—Nadi Shodhanam

a

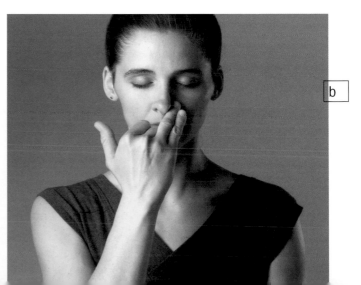

b

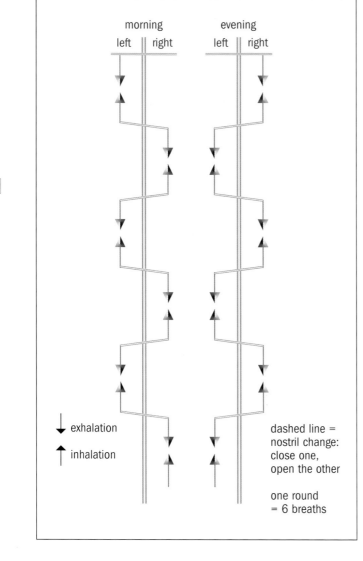

Nadi Shodhanam Breathing Patterns

morning

left right

evening

left right

↓ exhalation

↑ inhalation

dashed line =
nostril change:
close one,
open the other

one round
= 6 breaths

194

PATTERN FOR NADI SHODHANAM

There are a number of patterns for alternating the breath in the nostrils—some simple, and some complex. In the following method the flow is alternated with each full breath, and so it is easy to remember and monitor.

Yoga breathing exercises frequently begin with an exhalation. This is both symbolic and practical. Symbolically, it reminds us that we must prepare ourselves by emptying wastes and impurities. Practically, the exhalation is a cleansing breath and readies the lungs and nervous system for the inhalation, which is energizing.

The maxim "right at night" is an easy way to remember which side to begin on. At night, begin with an exhalation on the right side. In the morning, begin by exhaling through the left nostril. The midday practice pattern is determined by identifying which nostril is active (dominant) and which passive (non-dominant) at the time of practice, and exhaling on the passive side first.

THE TECHNIQUE

► Sit with your head, neck, and trunk erect so that your spine is balanced and steady and you can breathe freely. Gently close your eyes.

► Breathe diaphragmatically. Let each exhalation and inhalation be the same length—smooth, slow, and relaxed. Do not allow the breath to be forced or jerky. With practice, the length of the breath will increase.

► To begin the practice, close one nostril, then exhale and inhale smoothly and completely through the other. The inhalation and exhalation are of equal length and there is no sense of forcing the breath.

► Now alternate sides, completing one full breath on the opposite side.

► Continue alternating between the nostrils until you have completed a full round of the practice (3 breaths on each side, for a total of 6 breaths). Then lower your hand and breathe gently and smoothly through both nostrils. For a deeper practice, complete two more rounds. (Note: When practicing three rounds in one sitting, the second of the three rounds begins on the opposite nostril, and the pattern of alternation is therefore the reverse of rounds one and three.)

► Lower your hand and bring your attention to the breath flowing in the nostril that feels more open. Relax and attend to the sensation there for a number of breaths. Next, shift your attention to the breath in the more passive nostril. Keep your focus there for a longer time (you may find that the nostril opens). Again, simply attend to the flow of the breath.

▶ Finally, merge these two streams in your awareness, sensing the breath as if it is flowing from the base of the nose to the point between the eyebrows in one single, central stream. Let this focus become relaxed and one-pointed. Follow the breath, allowing your thoughts to come and go without disturbing your attention.

HINTS AND CAUTIONS

Nadi shodhanam is in many ways the most important of all pranayama practices. In the beginning it should be done twice a day—usually morning and evening. As part of a complete yoga practice session it is performed following postures and relaxation, and prior to meditation. Wait at least three hours after eating a meal before the practice, half an hour after liquids.

Do not practice channel purification if you are tired and cannot concentrate. Don't practice when you have a headache, when you are restless and agitated, or during periods of fever. Persons with a seizure disorder should not practice alternate nostril breathing. If noises in the head develop, discontinue the practice.

Developing a Pranayama Practice

Any of the techniques in this chapter might be the focus of practice, and a balanced pranayama routine can be developed that includes all of them. The nasal wash cleanses the upper respiratory tracts; the complete breath refreshes you when you are tired; agni sara is used to tone and strengthen the abdomen; kapalabhati works from the navel center upward, cleansing the lungs and invigorating energies; channel purification balances the entire system of energy, preparing it for relaxation and meditation, and leading to a calm and joyful state of mind.

Here is a practice routine that includes all the breathing techniques presented in this chapter.

A Practice Routine

Daily nasal wash.

Ten repetitions of agni sara.

One set of eleven repetitions of kapalabhati.

The complete breath at the outset of asana practice or in the late afternoon, following work.

One round of channel purification (morning and evening).

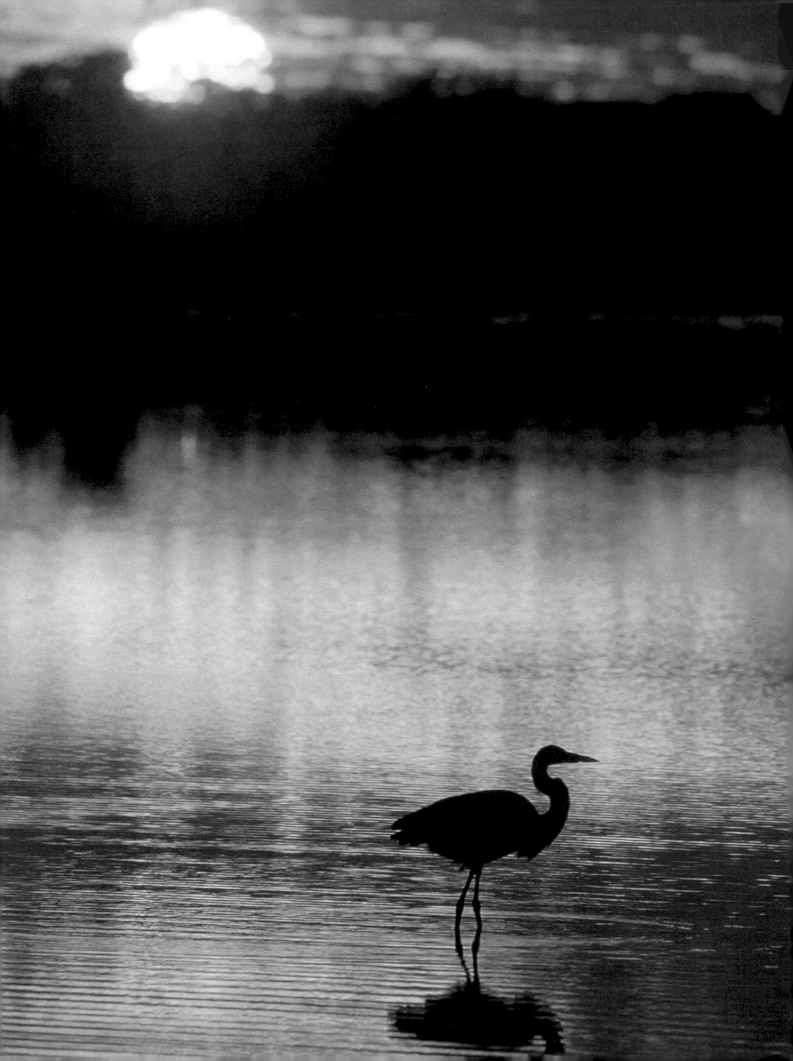

CHAPTER EIGHT

RELAXATION

Within creation are held in balance
the three realms of body, mind, and spirit.
—— *Rig Veda*

BENEATH the ups and downs of everyday life there is a profound state of balance. By resting for brief periods in that state we create a resilient and stable mind even in the face of stress. That is why each of us, on a deep level, craves relaxation—it revives our confidence and reawakens a sense of self-control. Yoga relaxation exercises quiet the senses and lead us beneath the restless surface of the mind. Through relaxation we restore a sense of inner harmony.

Relaxation exercises form the bridge between hatha yoga and the more subtle levels of self-awareness found in meditation. Each asana session ends with a 10–15 minute period of systematic relaxation, and this allows time for the mind and body to assimilate the benefits of the poses that have been completed. During relaxation the experience of the postures reverberates through muscles and other soft tissue, forming new patterns of internal sensation and new pathways for movement. Asanas and breath training are primarily designed to work with the body and nervous system; relaxation is a tool for calming the senses and mind.

Relaxation and meditation are actually stages in a continuous process. They are allied practices in the yoga system, but in order to give them adequate attention we have addressed them in two separate chapters. This chapter is devoted to relaxation; in the following chapter you will learn how meditation practices continue the journey inward. In effect, relaxation is like the roots and stem of a plant that blossoms in meditation. Relaxation exercises prepare the body and mind for meditation and lead to it gracefully. They may also be practiced by themselves simply for refreshment and rejuvenation, because relaxation is an essential tool for reducing fatigue and maintaining good health. Whenever you feel tired, distracted, or unable to focus, they can help.

STAGES OF PRACTICE

The process of relaxation and meditation progresses in five stages:
Stage One: Stillness
Stage Two: Diaphragmatic breathing
Stage Three: Systematic relaxation
Stage Four: Breath awareness in the nostrils
Stage Five: Mantra

The first three of these stages constitute relaxation practice—they still the body, relax and free the breath, and culminate in a formal relaxation technique. Stages four and five, the subject of the next chapter, are meditative practices. They refine concentration and ultimately allow attention to rest in a pure, mental focus. Together, the five stages are the foundation for relaxed self-awareness. Memorize the sequence now. When you close your eyes to begin your practice, you will find it helpful to have this framework in place.

The five stages flow from one to the other, overlap to some degree, and lead inward with increasing momentum. They are arranged from outer to inner—from physical self-awareness to the mind. They form a natural channel that will bring you to a vibrant, yet calm, center of consciousness. From there you will be able to witness the activity of the body and mind and at the same time remain relaxed and self-aware.

THE RELAXATION POSTURE

Relaxation practices are learned lying down. The primary posture is the corpse pose. In the corpse pose the force of gravity affects the body differently than it does in upright poses. For example, in a standing posture the heart must work against gravity to pump blood to the head and return blood from the feet; in the corpse pose the horizontal plane of the body makes the work of the heart easier and relieves muscle fatigue that results from maintaining an upright posture.

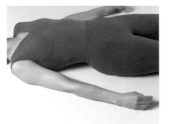
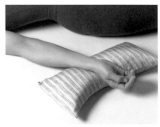

The Corpse Pose

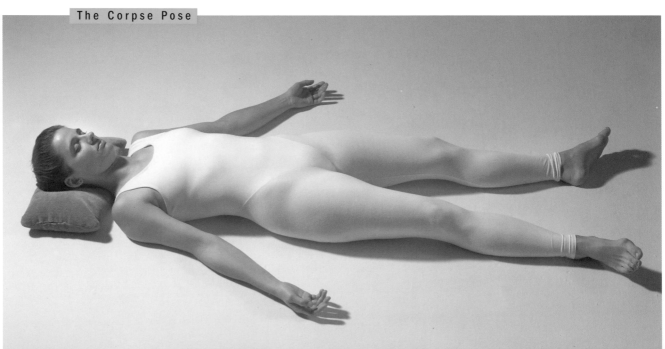

HINTS AND GUIDELINES

Paying attention to a few details can make the corpse pose more effective and comfortable.

▶ Empty the bladder before practice.

▶ Do not use a bed or couch for relaxation, but lie on a flat carpeted or padded surface.

▶ Use a thin cushion to support the head and neck— one filled with buckwheat hulls is excellent for this purpose, as it is cooling and can be shaped to the contour of the neck. However, any thin cushion can be used. The cushion bolsters the spine and relieves discomfort at the back of the head. Yoga adepts also tell us that a slightly raised head affects subtle energies in the body during relaxation, preventing heart problems.

▶ Lie with the body flat, the weight evenly distributed.

▶ Take care that the spine is not bent or rolled to either side.

▶ Make sure that the legs are slightly apart, and the arms rest alongside the body.

▶ If comfortable, turn the palms up. (To do this it may help to slide the shoulder blades slightly underneath the back, toward the spine.)

The corpse pose is a comfortable posture for most people, but a few minor adjustments can prevent unnecessary strain.

▶ Don't be too concerned if the hands roll toward the body, or even turn downward. Simply let the arms find a restful position.

▶ If discomfort in the lower back increases, try placing a folded blanket under your knees. The blanket can be rolled to any height. If a blanket is not available, raise your knees and lean them against one another.

▶ It may help to place a thin cushion under each hand if the elbows do not fully straighten with ease.

▶ Metabolism slows during relaxation, so cover yourself with a blanket or shawl to prevent a chill.

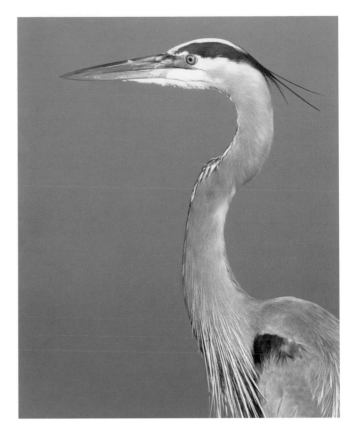

STAGE ONE: STILLNESS

Nature reminds us of the importance of being still. The tall, slender crane can remain motionless for long periods of time, and because of this it has become a striking symbol of stillness. But when fishing, its stillness is charged with anticipation for the impending thrust; and when sleeping, its stillness lacks awareness and energy. When the crane is standing quietly, however— attentive and serene—its stillness is like yoga relaxation.

Neither poised for action, nor sleepy and lethargic, the stillness of yogic relaxation is marked by quiet observation of the body. This is a state that cannot be cultivated with force. In fact, making an effort to be still creates energy that is contrary to relaxation.

The way to achieve a restful stillness is deceptively simple. Just recline comfortably and let time pass as you allow your breath to flow freely out and in. Soon you will feel stillness rising within you. And if you continue resting patiently you will find that this sense of stillness emerges from a great, unseen depth. It will hold and support you, and you can rest in it.

Staying Awake

It is easy to fall asleep while reclining during relaxation exercises. To remain alert:

▶ Deepen your breath.
▶ Firmly maintain awareness of the flow of the breath.
▶ Do not practice relaxation immediately after meals.
▶ Do a few yoga stretches just before practice.
▶ Get enough sleep at night.
▶ If necessary, practice sitting up—leaning against a wall.

PROBLEMS

Occasionally restlessness makes the beginning stage of relaxation difficult. When the mind and body are unable to settle down, a few stretches, a brief walk, or a splash of water on the face and neck are useful preparations for relaxing. The technique of tensing and relaxing, described later in the chapter, can also help.

It is also common to experience twitches and other small muscle spasms during the first few minutes of relaxation. These often occur in the early stages of sleep as well, but are rarely cause for concern—the body is releasing tensions and will soon quiet down.

Overly stimulating foods and the body's own stress hormones can be another cause of discomfort. Caffeine is notorious for agitating the mind, and other foods such as sugar and alcohol also create restlessness and mental tension. When the mind is imbalanced by something you have eaten, it may be necessary to wait for the discomfort to pass before relaxing.

The stress response, resulting in the release of adrenaline or cortisol into the bloodstream, also causes agitation, and these biochemicals may take many minutes, or even hours, to wend their way through the body. Breathing can help calm jangled nerves, and a walk or a hatha yoga session is a good way to de-escalate heightened energy. Of course, problems with food or stress remind us that good lifestyle choices are wise investments of energy. For more about lifestyle, there are other useful suggestions in chapter 10 to help reduce overall tension levels.

With practice, a restful stillness can develop relatively quickly—in just a minute or two. Then sounds from the outer environment come and go without creating a disturbance, and the body settles into a fathomless sense of inner stillness, where it rests. This state is highly reassuring. It provides stability and a foundation for continuing further in the relaxation process.

STAGE TWO: RELAXING THE BREATH

At the outset of relaxation practice, breathing takes place at the edges of awareness. As the relaxation period continues, however, attention turns more and more toward the breath. And finally, its rhythmic pulsing becomes the primary focus of attention. During this stage, awareness remains centered on the breath as it systematically cleanses and then nourishes.

But watching the breath can prove deceptively challenging. In the beginning the mind is active, and thoughts move more rapidly than the breath. In fact, the speed of the breath feels painfully slow compared to the speed of thinking. Attending to the breath may even seem boring. Fortunately, however, the process of watching the breath influences the mind, and with time, the frenetic pace of thinking is gradually relieved. A calm focus develops. Each exhalation feels relaxing, and each inhalation feels nourishing.

SHAPING THE BREATH

As the mind tracks the breath it gradually shapes it and at the same time relieves the tensions that distort its normal flow. But this process requires time and experience to perfect. When we try too hard to breathe correctly we usually manage to introduce new tensions. On the other hand, if we give the breath too little attention it remains automatic and outside our awareness. Our goal is to let the breath flow with a relaxed effort.

Once diaphragmatic breathing is established, we can turn our attention to the five basic qualities of breathing: we develop a breath that is deep, smooth, even, without sound, and without pause. During this phase of breath awareness the mind calmly scans for difficulties, unblocking tension and allowing the flow of the breath to unfold with each passing moment.

ALLOWING THE BODY TO BREATHE

As relaxation deepens, conscious involvement with breathing gradually changes. A state of relaxed awareness in which the breath flows effortlessly of its own accord replaces the endeavor to shape the breath. Still absorbed in the sensations of this unbroken flow, the mind relaxes.

Breathing, of course, continues on its circular journey whether we pay attention to it or not. In a sense, our lengthy process of breath training has only brought us back to where we began: the automatic flow of the breath. But now the quality of the breath has been improved, and awareness of its flow can be maintained at will.

At first it can be disconcerting when conscious efforts to breathe are relaxed. It is easy to become self-conscious and again "take charge." Gradually, however, the joy of watching the breath outweighs the joy of commanding it, and relaxation deepens. Then each breath flows naturally into the next without pause, and the restless energies of the mind and body become quiet.

STAGE THREE: SYSTEMATIC RELAXATION

Stillness and relaxed breathing provide a solid foundation for the third stage of relaxation practice: a methodical relaxation technique. Below you will find three different methods to try. They vary in their approach, but all lead to a deep state of relaxation.

METHOD ONE: SYSTEMATIC MUSCLE RELAXATION

This is the relaxation technique you will probably use more than any other. Here, awareness travels from the head to the toes, and then from the toes back to the head, as if making a procession through the body. At each of the areas listed below, muscle tension is relaxed while natural, diaphragmatic breathing is maintained. During the downward descent through the body the attention rests briefly at four places—the nose, the fingertips, the heart, and the toes—while the focus shifts almost entirely to breath awareness. Then the procession continues.

Pausing for breath awareness during systematic muscle relaxation can seem unnecessary or time-consuming, but it is an important component in the process of relaxation. Wherever mental attention is focused, prana, or energy, is also awakened. Pausing for breath awareness is a means of relaxing and energizing the body and systematically enhancing the flow of prana.

After the excursion through the body has been completed, breath awareness is again sustained for 10 breaths or longer with the focus on the whole body. This completes the exercise.

Here is the order of progression through the muscles. (You may wish to record the list slowly in your own voice.) Travel to each of the following areas of your body, resting your awareness at the:

- Crown of the head
- Forehead and temples
- Eyebrows, eyelids, and eyes
- Nose (attention rests at the nose, breathing out and in with awareness 2–4 times)
- Cheeks and jaw
- Mouth and chin
- Throat
- Sides and back of the neck
- Shoulders
- Upper arms; lower arms
- Hands; fingers
- Fingertips (attention rests at the fingertips; inhale as if the breath flows down to the fingertips, then exhale up and out the nostrils, 2–4 times)
- Fingers; hands; arms
- Shoulders
- Chest and rib cage around the back to the spine
- Heart center (not the physical heart, but the center of energy between the breasts at the base of the sternum and deep to the surface of the chest); inhale as if breathing down to the heart center; then exhale up and out the nostrils, 2–4 times
- Abdomen
- Sides, lower back
- Hips, buttocks
- Upper legs; lower legs
- Feet
- Toes (attention rests at the toes; inhale as if breathing down to the toes, then exhale up and out the nostrils, 2–4 times)
- Now, return upward in reverse order without pausing for breath awareness at any of the points.
- Finish with 10 or more relaxed breaths, breathing as if the whole body breathes. Relax your body, breath, and mind.

202

Systematic Relaxation in a Nutshell

- Establish stillness and diaphragmatic breathing.
- Start from the crown of the head, traveling down through the body and back to the crown.
- Going downward, pause for breath awareness at the points noted.
- At the end of the exercise, breathe 10 or more times as if the whole body breathes.
- The entire exercise takes 10–12 minutes.

Notes on Practice

The apparent similarity between relaxation exercises and hypnotic inductions sometimes raises questions. There are similarities in technique, it is true, but the purpose as well as the inner technique of relaxation exercises is different from hypnosis. In hypnosis the mind receives suggestions—either from the hypnotist or from oneself in the form of auto-suggestion—which the subject willingly accepts.

Relaxation techniques are at once more simple and more subtle. As awareness moves through the body the yoga practitioner is not making suggestions to the muscles. Nor is relaxation induced by hypnotic trance. During systematic muscle relaxation you are learning to give relaxed attention to each area, and this allows muscles to release tension and to rest in whatever way feels natural. In other words, the point is not to induce relaxation, but to relax. Experienced yoga practitioners often remind us that we are already hypnotized by the expectations and suggestions of the world. They say that yoga is a technique for awakening awareness, not for putting it to sleep with more suggestions!

METHOD TWO: TENSION/RELAXATION

Some students have difficulty bringing awareness to a specific area of the body and resting it there in a systematic muscle relaxation. They may find it difficult to identify that area, or feelings of agitation and restlessness may intrude, resulting in an overwhelming desire to move the body. One way to address these problems is to practice a tension/relaxation exercise.

In tension/relaxation a brief period of relaxed breath awareness once more sets the stage for progressive movement through the body. This time specific areas are first tensed and then relaxed, and the noticeable contrast in the state of the muscles helps to develop body awareness and reduce the effects of restlessness. In this exercise tension is created and directed in an orderly way, first by slowly moving into it, usually in coordination with the breath; then by holding it briefly while practicing breath awareness; and finally by releasing the tension slowly, again in coordination with the breath.

During this exercise one must pay attention to the capacity of the body and mind. If the body begins to tremble it is important to reduce the tension until the shaking ends. (Shaking is a sign that the nervous system is being strained.) Similarly, when the tension becomes so absorbing that breath awareness is lost, the attention should be brought back to the breath. Maintain a relaxed flow of breathing throughout the exercise.

Caution: Tension/relaxation exercises should not be practiced by persons with hypertension (high blood pressure). Consult with your doctor.

Here is the sequence for practice. (Again, you may wish to record it.)

► Rest comfortably, developing a relaxed flow of breathing.
► Inhaling, raise the eyebrows, tensing the forehead; hold the tension for 1–2 relaxed breaths; release with an exhalation.
► Exhaling, squeeze the facial muscles inward as if focusing at the nose; hold the tension for 1–2 relaxed breaths; release with an inhalation.
► Exhaling, twist the head to the right; without pausing, inhale and return the head to the center. Exhaling, twist the head to the left; without pausing, inhale and return the head to the center.
► Let the head and neck rest and become still.
► Turn the palms toward the floor. Exhaling, press downward from the shoulders to the fingers; hold the tension for 1–2 relaxed breaths; release with an inhalation.
► Turn the palms up once more and make a fist with the palms. Inhaling, tense the fists and arms; hold the tension for 1–2 relaxed breaths; release the tension with an exhalation.
► Let the arms and shoulders release to the floor and become still.
► Inhaling, slowly expand the chest and upper back; without pausing, exhale and relax the chest and upper back. Rest and breathe.
► Exhaling, slowly contract the abdomen; without pausing, inhale and relax the abdomen. Rest and breathe.
► Exhaling, tense the buttocks; hold the tension for 1–2 relaxed breaths; release the tension slowly with an inhalation.
► Roll the legs so that the kneecaps face upward, and point the toes away from the body. Exhaling, tense the legs and feet; hold the tension for 1–2 relaxed breaths; release the tension slowly with an inhalation. (If the arch of the foot begins to cramp, soften the foot extension.) Rest the legs.
► Roll the legs so that the kneecaps face upward, and pull the toes toward the body. Inhaling, tense the feet and legs; hold the tension for 1–2 relaxed breaths; exhaling, release the tension slowly.
► Rest the whole body.

► Now tense the whole body at once. Again roll the legs so that the kneecaps face upward, and point the toes away from the body. Turn the palms toward the floor. Exhaling, tense the legs and feet, tense the abdomen, tense the arms and shoulders against the floor, and squeeze the facial muscles inward as if focusing at the nose; without stopping the breath, inhale and release the tension through the whole body. Relax and breathe.

► Again tense the whole body, this time on an inhalation. Roll the legs so that the kneecaps face upward, and pull the toes toward the body. Make a fist with the hands. Inhaling, tense the feet and legs, expand the chest and upper back, tense the arms, and squeeze the face; without stopping the breath, exhale and release the tension through the whole body.

► Allow your entire body to rest. Breathe out and in, feeling the breath cleanse as it flows out, and nourish as it flows in.

► This exercise can be followed by systematic relaxation, or you can simply lie resting, breathing as if the whole body breathes. Exhaling, let the breath seem to release tensions and wastes from the entire body. Inhaling, let the breath seem to nourish every cell and tissue.

► Remain resting and quietly breathing for 5–10 breaths. Watch the breath—relaxing your body, breath, and mind.

METHOD THREE:
POINT-TO-POINT BREATHING

In the third relaxation technique, point-to-point breathing, the breath plays an even greater role in creating a rested and relaxed focus. This is a wonderfully soothing exercise, and is especially useful when the mind is fatigued or when the body feels lethargic and heavy.

In point-to-point breathing imagine that with each exhalation awareness and the breath travel downward

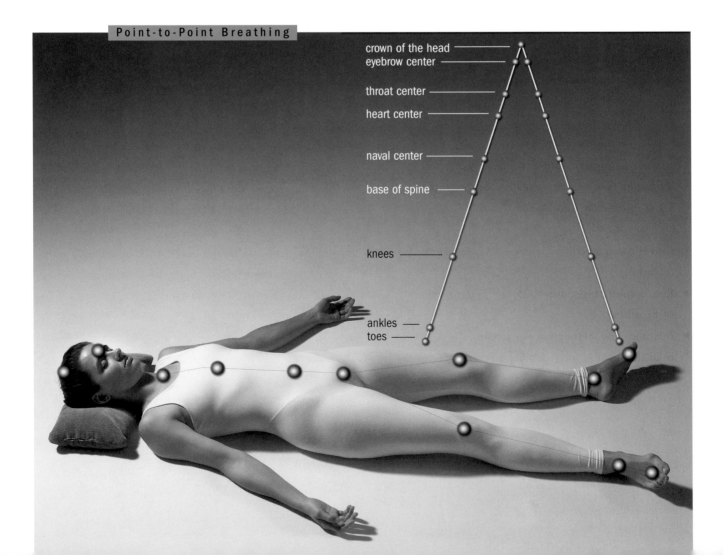

Point-to-Point Breathing

crown of the head
eyebrow center

throat center

heart center

naval center

base of spine

knees

ankles
toes

together through the body, from the crown of the head to one of eight points, before returning to the crown with the inhalation. The points start with the toes of the feet and move progressively upward. After completing all eight levels of breathing in an ascending order, the pattern is reversed and the breath is gradually moved back down to the toes.

Throughout this exercise it is important to let the breath flow smoothly, without pausing between breaths. And it is important to remember that even though the distance your awareness travels in the body becomes shorter, the breath nonetheless remains deep and relaxed. With regular practice this will result in a refined breath that flows slowly but without jerkiness. Concentration will improve, and at the conclusion of the exercise the entire body will feel refreshed. Here is the sequence for practice:

- Rest in the corpse pose, allowing the body to become still.
- Establish relaxed, diaphragmatic breathing.
- Observing your breathing, exhale as if the breath is flowing from the crown of your head down to your toes. Inhale back to the crown of the head. Repeat 2–5 times here and at all subsequent points except as noted.
- Exhale from the crown down to the level of the ankles, and inhale back to the crown.
- Exhale down to the level of the knees.
- Exhale down to the level of the base of the spine.
- Exhale down to the level of the navel center.
- Exhale down to the level of the heart center.
- Exhale down to the level of the throat.
- Exhale down to the level of the eyebrow center. Breathe back and forth between the crown and the eyebrow center, refining the breath and resting, 5–10 times.
- Now reverse the order and descend, first to the throat center, then to the heart center, to the navel center, and so on, until you return to the toes.

- Finish by breathing as if the whole body breathes. Let the exhalation flow downward as if through the soles of the feet and on to infinity. Inhaling, breathe as if the breath were a wave flowing upward through the body and the crown of the head and on to infinity. Sense that you are lying in the center of a wave of energy and bliss. Let your breathing remain deep, and watch the breath as you relax your body, breath, and mind.

In the End

We have described three methods for systematic relaxation. No matter which of the three techniques you use, spend a few minutes resting after it has been completed—quietly observing your body, breath, and mind. When you are finished, stretch in whatever way is comfortable, cover your eyes with your palms, open your eyes slowly, and remove your hands. Finally, roll to your side and come back to a sitting position. If you are using the relaxation technique as a preparation for meditating, then you will take your meditation seat and continue. Otherwise, this completes your session.

Relaxation techniques can be used in many ways. Take a break from a busy schedule by relaxing in the mid-afternoon. For a short period of relaxing breath awareness, close your eyes while sitting at your desk or in your living room. Before giving a speech or performing in some other way, find a corner in which to lie down and relax. But, above all, use a relaxation technique once or twice every day to maintain a center of calmness and well-being that will reflect in everything you do. Relaxation is a skill that soon becomes part of the fabric of life. And as you will see in the next chapter, it is a pathway that leads still further inward to the quietest recesses of your being.

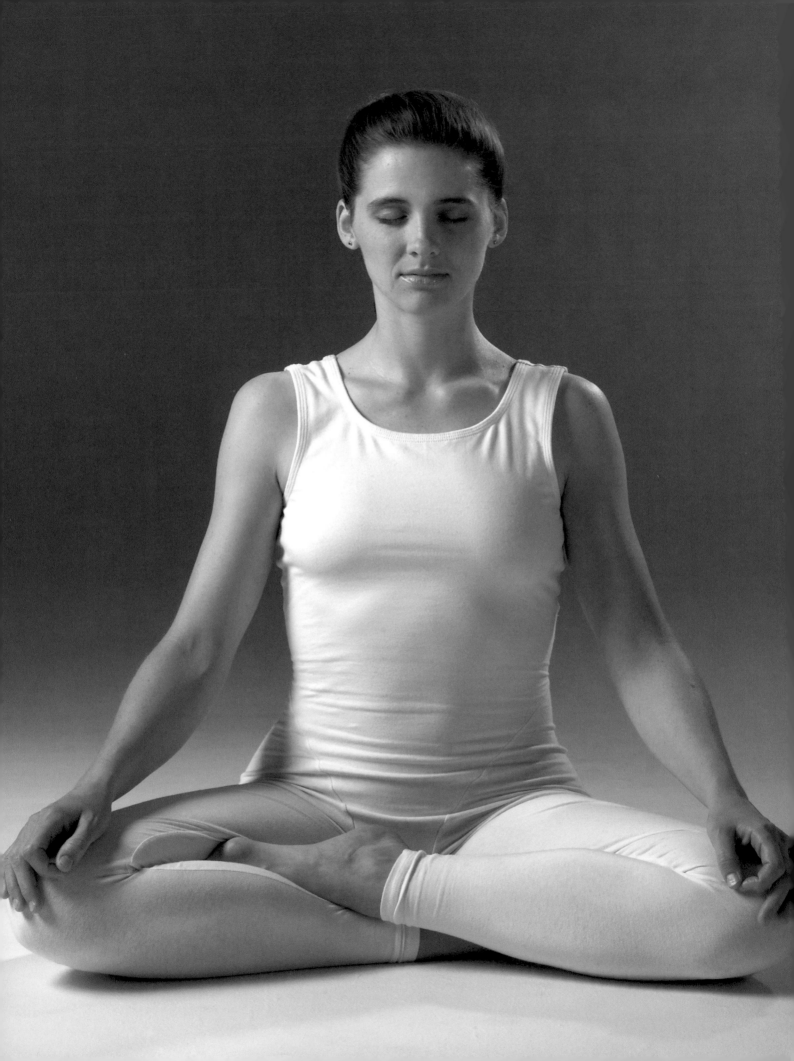

CHAPTER NINE

MEDITATION

> Meditation gives you what nothing else can give you:
> it introduces you to yourself.
> ——— *Swami Rama*

YOGA is a journey toward self-awareness. On this journey relaxation skills help us gather the disparate energies of the body and mind and focus them internally. Then mental distractions intrude with less intensity, and a sense of inner flexibility and calmness develops. Relaxation also prepares the personality for a still more interior practice: meditation. Through meditation we can safely enter the quiet and inward places of the mind and heart.

"The mind alone is the cause of bondage and of liberation," the yogis tell us, because long ago they observed that the mind is like a lens through which we experience both the inner and outer worlds—it is the source of distress as well as the means for illumination.

This insight led to meditative practices that incline the mind toward clarity and encourage self-awareness. They calm its turbulence, and through their steadying, purifying, and harmonizing influence they help us discover the true nature of the self.

THE MIND IN MEDITATION

We all know that whenever we become over-involved with the flow of outer experience our inner balance is disturbed. Our natural serenity is replaced by attachments and agitation. On the other hand, when our inner life is balanced the forces of attachment are weakened, the mind becomes calm, and there is a clear field into which the light and energy of the self can radiate. We are composed and naturally joyful. When we are fully anchored in this state, the sage Patanjali tells us, "the self abides in its own nature." When we can learn to make our mind still we will find our own true self shining beneath the disturbance.

Meditation offers a way to accomplish this. Like watching the flow of a river from its bank, a meditator learns to maintain a watchful, inner stance, and from that perspective the stream of outward events can be experienced while the meditator remains centered and relaxed. This process gradually leads to a deeper core of self-awareness. Thus meditation is both a way of enjoying life more fully and a way of gaining self-knowledge— direct, immediate, and without distortion.

Because meditation engages directly with the mind, it lies at the heart of raja yoga, the royal path. In fact Svatmarama, a great teacher of hatha yoga, maintained that the purpose of hatha was "solely for the attainment of the royal path." Postures, breath training, and relaxation techniques, he said, all serve the more inward goal of meditation. Many centuries earlier the sage Vasishtha had taught his beloved student Rama: "The self is not realized by any means other than meditation."

HOW TO MEDITATE

At the heart of meditation practice are two inseparable skills. The first is concentration, the ability to rest your attention on a focus. The other is mindfulness, the ability to observe your personality with compassionate detachment. These two work together to create a clear and one-pointed mind.

Meditation does not require a change in religious faith or the endorsement of a particular dogma. Its spiritual aspect is universal; it can be practiced by people of all faiths or by those who have no formal religion at all.

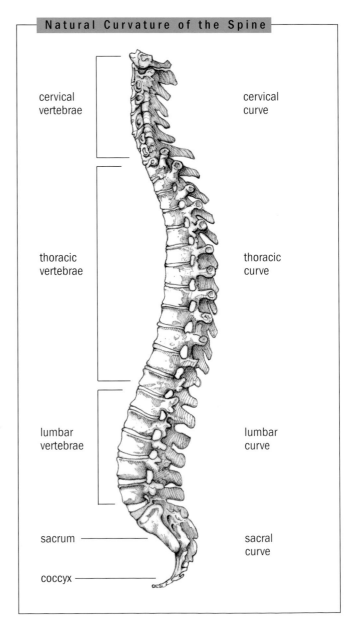

Natural Curvature of the Spine

cervical vertebrae

cervical curve

thoracic vertebrae

thoracic curve

lumbar vertebrae

lumbar curve

sacrum

sacral curve

coccyx

Here are the steps in the process:

- Develop a steady, comfortable sitting posture.
- Use the processes of stillness, diaphragmatic breathing, and systematic relaxation learned in the preceding chapters to set the stage for meditation.
- Create a relaxed focus on the breath.
- Rest your awareness on a mantra, or inner sound.
- Practice mindfulness—the act of compassionately witnessing, but not identifying with, your body, nervous system, and mind.

DEVELOPING A SITTING POSTURE

Meditation begins with preparation. Students do not simply sit down and enter the deepest state. There are transitions to be observed. Just as a musician prepares for a performance by playing scales and familiar passages, so does the meditator begin with personal rituals that establish a mood.

- The seat is arranged.
- Constricting clothing is loosened.
- The legs and arms are brought gently into place.
- The eyes are closed.
- The posture is fine-tuned.

Only then does the familiar inner process begin to unfold.

Because physical discomfort and mental chatter are intertwined, the first step in calming the mind is to stabilize and quiet the body. But anyone who has tried to sit perfectly still for any length of time can testify that it is not easy to find a stable and comfortable sitting pose.

The spine is not perfectly straight. Its natural curvature reduces the likelihood of injury and fatigue, and adds resiliency to the skeletal structure. But this means that to sit steadily and comfortably for any length of time the head, neck, and trunk must be aligned directly over the base of the spine. Sitting straight actually means aligning and balancing the spine along a vertical axis ascending toward the skull. Distortions are not only uncomfortable and destabilizing, they also block the flow of energy at subtle levels.

Sitting straight is not as simple as it sounds. Most of us have habitual muscular tensions, stiffness, and/or weakness in the spine, the pelvis, the legs, or the shoulder girdle that hinder our efforts to sit straight. For example, if the shoulders are rounded and pulled in toward the chest it is difficult to straighten the upper back and open the chest.

Another common problem is pelvic alignment. A steady, stable posture requires that we sit squarely on the base of the spine. If the lower back is stiff or if the hamstrings or inner thigh muscles are tight, these muscles tug on the pelvis, distorting the natural curve in the lower back: the lower back collapses and the upper back rounds forward to counterbalance the feeling of falling backward.

The pelvic foundation can also be distorted by over-arching the lower back in an attempt to sit up straight. This thrusts the pelvis forward, creating tension in the spine as well as in the hips, thighs, and neck. It often leads to pain in the muscular attachments below the shoulder blades as well.

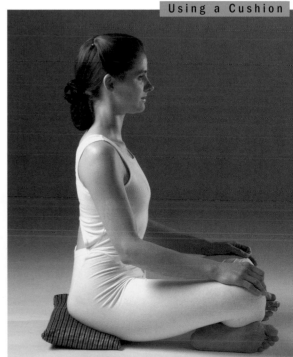

Using a Cushion

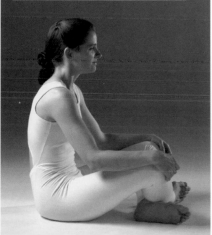

Collapsed Lower Back

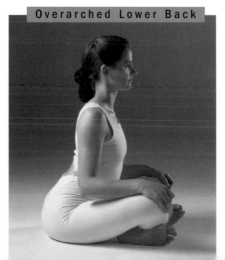

Overarched Lower Back

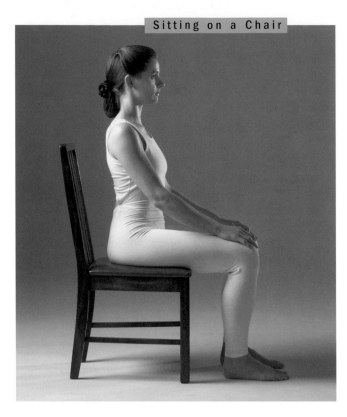

A simple prop offers dramatic improvement for the collapsed lower back. Placing a cushion or a folded blanket under the buttocks elevates the base of the spine, compensating for limited flexibility and restoring the natural curve. To correct an overarched lower back, release unnecessary tension in the pelvis.

Regular work with hatha yoga postures improves alignment and comfort in the sitting poses by developing flexibility in the legs, hips, and spine; strengthening the lower back; opening the chest; and increasing self-awareness. But there is no need to put off your meditation practice until you have perfect flexibility and strength. There are a number of sitting postures which, when properly executed, keep the spine straight, the body comfortable, the subtle energies collected and directed, the breath steady and smooth, and the mind calm and clear. Here are four of them:

SITTING ON A CHAIR (MAITRYASANA)

Those whose knee, hip, or lower back flexibility is compromised by old injuries, arthritis, or other persistent conditions may find that sitting on a chair is the solution to establishing a steady and comfortable posture that keeps the spine straight. Our muscles are accustomed to sitting on chairs, so this pose makes no unusual demands on the knees and hips.

► Find a chair with a firm, flat surface. Sit forward on it with your knees straight out from the hips, feet flat on the floor and pointed forward. The height of the chair is an important consideration. It is useful in all the seated postures (except perhaps the easy pose) to have the hips slightly higher than the knees. Then the thighs slope gently downward, and strain in the legs is minimized. A cushion can be used to raise the height of the seat if necessary. If your feet aren't solidly on the floor, place a phone book or some other flat support under them.

► Close your eyes, press down through the base of the spine, and lift up through the top of the head.

► Lift your shoulders, roll them up and back, and then drop and relax them.

► Allow your hands to fall naturally on the thighs, and join the tips of the thumbs and forefingers. The chair doesn't create any difficulties for the body; it can be used by anyone who is not comfortable on the floor.

THE EASY POSE (SUKHASANA)

The chair is comfortable, but the linear support it provides to the base of the body is not as stable or grounded as the triangular foundation created by sitting cross-legged on the floor. The cross-legged poses have the additional advantage of drawing the legs and feet in toward the torso, which collects our energy and directs it inward. In addition to helping straighten the spine, bending the knees and crossing the legs create "locks," which have subtle but profound effects in the pelvis and lower back.

The easy pose is the cross-legged sitting posture that requires the least flexibility in the knees and hips.

▶ To assume the pose, sit on a cushion or folded blanket and cross the legs. If possible, allow each leg to rest on the opposite foot.

▶ Align the upper body and shoulders directly over the base of the spine and rest the hands on the thighs.

Experiment with different cushion heights until you feel comfortable. Make sure the cushion is not too soft. Firmness at the base of the spine is important not only for long-term support and comfort but also for stimulating and directing subtle energies.

Frequently the knees, hips, or back are irritated by sitting cross-legged in this pose for any extended length of time, and if you choose this posture for meditation you can relieve discomfort by placing a cushion or rolled blanket under the thigh and knee to support the joint and alleviate the stress. Remember, we are searching for both comfort and stability, and one follows the other. Even if only one leg is problematic for you, it is better to provide support under both legs—be careful not to disturb the symmetry of the pose by propping one knee too high.

THE AUSPICIOUS POSE (SVASTIKASANA)

The auspicious pose is more stable and collected than the easy pose because it folds the feet and legs more tightly together and closer to the torso. It also allows the thighs and the knees to rest on the floor, and positions the feet near the pubis. The tighter locks in the legs, however, require more hip, ankle, and knee flexibility than the easy pose.

▶ To assume the pose, place the sole of the left foot against the right thigh.

▶ Tuck the right foot between the left thigh and calf.

▶ You may pull the left foot up a little so that it is between the right thigh and calf. The ankles are crossed in front of the pubic bone and the feet are sandwiched between the opposite thighs and calves.

▶ Align the upper torso over the base of the spine, using a cushion at the base of the spine as necessary.

When the legs and ankles are locked in this pose the spine is naturally lifted, and the flow of energy in the legs is directed into the base of the spine. If you are comfortable in this posture you will feel your attention drawn inward and your mind quieted.

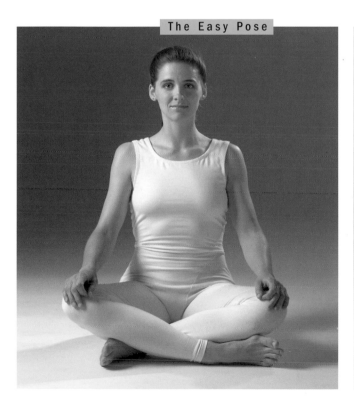

The Easy Pose

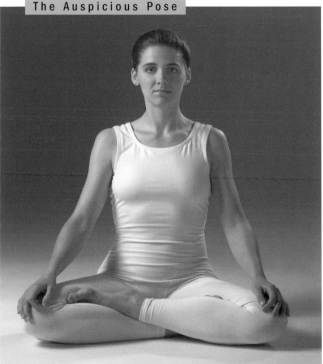

The Auspicious Pose

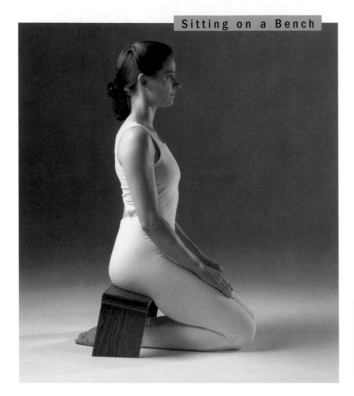

Sitting on a Bench

THE BENCH POSE

The bench pose provides an alternative for those who would like to sit on the floor but who have problems that prevent them from sitting cross-legged. Here the shins are resting on the floor, which makes this posture more stable than sitting on a chair. And while the bench pose is not as effective as the auspicious pose in drawing energy inward to the base of the spine, it does provide good support and lift to the spinal column.

Before you can sit in this pose you will need to purchase or make a bench with a slanted seat.

► First kneel, then place the bench over your thighs with the seat slanting downward toward your knees.

► Sit back on the seat, keeping your thighs parallel and straight out from the hips. The toes are turned inward and the heels are slightly farther apart.

► The height of the seat can be raised by placing a cushion under your buttocks. A folded towel or thin cushion under each ankle will relieve pressure there, if necessary.

► Once you are comfortable the hands may be rested on the upper thighs or nested together.

Regardless of which posture you choose for your meditation practice, perfecting your posture leads the body and mind into ever deeper states of stillness. A perfectly stable posture focuses the body in the same way that an object of concentration focuses the mind. All the energies flow in one direction; the posture is held effortlessly, and body awareness no longer impinges on the mind. You will also notice that the breath becomes stable and effortless—more regular, smooth, quiet, and subtle. Then you are ready to enter a phase of concentration in which the mind itself is ultimately the object of attention.

Guidelines for Practicing Meditation

► Practice once or twice every day at about the same time.

► Practice before meals, not after.

► Early morning, late afternoon, and before bedtime are good times for practice.

► Empty your bladder before practicing.

► Create a pleasant space for practice, one that is neither cluttered nor confined.

► Start with 10 minutes and increase the time gradually until you enjoy sitting for 30 minutes.

► Observe your mind's capacity and do not fight to sit longer.

► Reinforce your practice with reading and contemplation.

CONCENTRATION

The preliminary practices of stillness, diaphragmatic breathing, and relaxation are all forms of concentration. Physical stillness brings our attention to the sensations of the body and rests it there; diaphragmatic breathing narrows the focus, bringing awareness to the ceaseless flow of the breath; systematic relaxation further refines the focus by releasing deep muscle tensions and merging awareness of the body and breath into an experience of internal wholeness. These practices lead us progressively inward.

But to meditate we must shift our attention to an even more subtle dimension of personality: to the mind itself. By choosing an appropriate object for concentration we can calm the mind's habit of moving restlessly from one experience to another. And then we will know the mind as we have never known it before—observing and guiding its play of thoughts with a natural sense of inner detachment.

Two objects for concentration are commonly used; each furthers the inward movement of awareness. The first is the touch of the breath in the nostrils, which is a highly refined sensory experience. As you focus on the sensations of the breath the other senses are rested, their activity is naturally quieted, and they withdraw. This withdrawal of the senses leads in turn to an even more inward concentration: focus on a mantra, a mental sound. Let's look at each of these stages in detail.

THE BREATH IN THE NOSTRILS

The touch of the breath is delicate—it would be difficult to produce another sensation as gentle as the soft touch of the air in the nose. When you exhale, the breath is warm and moist (humidified by the lungs); the inhalation is cool and dry (the condition of external air). You will need to make only a most modest effort to experience these two sensations. They are inherent in the act of breathing and can be brought to awareness any time you choose. Try the following exercise:

▶ Sit in your meditative pose and make yourself comfortable.

▶ Close your eyes and turn your attention to the touch of the breath in the nostrils, observing it continuously for several minutes. Feel the cool touch of the inhalation, and the warm touch of the exhalation. As the breath changes direction do not lose your focus—this is a time when it is easy for the mind to wander off. Relax and follow the breath carefully, sensing each inhalation and exhalation as well as each transition between breaths.

▶ As this process continues you may find that your mind oscillates between relaxation and restlessness. It may decide that you have focused on the sensation of the breath long enough. It may wander off, seeking pleasure from some other activity. It may not see any benefit or derive any exciting experience from the practice. Through all the mind's distractions your task is to remain relaxed, letting the thoughts come and go.

▶ When your awareness does wander, gently bring it back to the breath. Do not criticize yourself or expect your mind to stop thinking. Simply continue with the practice until even the effort to concentrate begins to relax.

▶ Learn to rest in a silence that coexists with the inner dialogue of your mind. Some meditators describe this as similar to the experience of slipping beneath the surface of the waves when you are snorkeling or diving. The waves have not disappeared, but they have lost their power to toss you about. Continue with your practice every day, fixing your attention on the breath and then relaxing your effort.

Breath awareness will lead you to a remarkably relaxing state of mind. Your concentration will be serene, you will be attentive to your mental processes in a soft and yielding manner, and when the mind becomes distracted a natural inwardness will bring you back to your center of awareness. This is meditative concentration.

MANTRA

The next step in meditation training is to unite the touch of the breath with a mantra, a sound which takes the form of a word or group of words. The two syllables of the Sanskrit word *mantra* give important clues about its meaning. The first syllable *(man)* is the verb "to think" (and is the source of the English word "man," a creature who thinks). The second syllable *(tra)* is related to the verb "to protect, guide, or lead." Thus a mantra is a thought that protects, guides, and leads. A mantra can be chanted aloud, or recited quietly, but it is most effective when it is allowed to reverberate in the mind without being externalized. The internal repetition calms thinking and refines concentration.

S o h a m

Each student is first taught a mantra that can be coordinated with breathing: the mantra *soham* (pronounced "so-hum"). It is said that *soham* is the natural sound of the breath and that, simply by breathing, everyone is unconsciously reciting this mantra throughout the day. But bringing *soham* to awareness within the mind, yogis say, makes the inaudible vibration of this mantra audible so that it may be used as a resting place during meditation. Try this exercise:

▶ Sit in your meditation posture and gradually bring your attention to the breath touching the inside of the nostrils.

▶ Relaxing your effort, allow your thoughts to come and go without disturbing your attention.

▶ Now, during the inhalation, let the sound *"so…"* resonate in the mind. During the exhalation, hear the sound *"hum…"* in the mind. Each sound lasts through the length of the entire breath. The sounds are not made audible. They quietly reverberate in the mind, flowing along with the natural movement of the two breaths.

▶ Don't make the mistake of altering your breathing in order to accommodate the pace of the two sounds

in the mind. Even though the mantra *soham* is indeed calming, and could be imprinted upon the breath, it is much better to let the breath flow at its natural pace and to hear the two sounds of the mantra as if they were accompanying it. Very soon, your breathing will relax and the sound itself will calm and center you.

As with mantras in general, there is no one precise translation for the sound *soham*. We can gain a sense of its significance, however, if we remember that the central theme of yoga is the journey toward the self.

Soham is a compound word, the union of the words *sah* and *aham* (the sound *so* is modified from the sound *sah*). *Sah* is the Sanskrit pronoun "that," but in this case "that" does not refer to a temporal object—it refers to our own pure self. The word *aham* is the personal pronoun "I"; it represents all the powers and forces that comprise the individual personality.

When these two words are combined they may be translated "I am That," affirming that deep within us is an identity that transcends the temporary pleasures, sorrows, and expectations of the external world. The mantra *soham* reminds us of that identity and helps us center ourselves and create a relationship with that deeper self.

The sound of the mantra *soham* (or any mantra, for that matter) expresses literally an inward energy that leads to an inward state of consciousness. The actual meaning of the mantra is the new perspective which it gradually unveils to those who recite it. Repeating its sound with dedication and openness to its energy invokes its guiding and nurturing potential.

But it is not necessary to have blind faith in the yoga tradition in order to practice the repetition of *soham*. All that is needed is a sense of respect and a genuine willingness to let the sound become the relaxed focus of your attention. That will allow the coordination of breath and sound to have its natural effect on the mind and personality.

How to Refine Your Concentration

In the process of refining your concentration there is a gradual transition from the focus on the breath in the nostrils to the focus on a mantra. This transition takes place in four stages:

▶ First rest your awareness on the breath in the nostrils with no mental sound.

▶ Next rest your awareness on the breath in the nostrils along with the sound of the breath *(soham)*.

▶ Then rest your awareness on the sound *soham* with only the merest awareness of the breath.

▶ Finally, rest your awareness on a personal mantra that transcends breath awareness.

A Personal Mantra

The mantra *soham* may be practiced by anyone. But many mantras used in yoga are given by a teacher to an individual student through a process of initiation. The mantra then becomes the student's personal mantra— a word or phrase revealed specifically to the teacher for the initiate during the process of giving the mantra. It is said that, following initiation, the energy of the mantra guides and protects the initiate.

Is there a basis for these beliefs? Yogis say there is. But perhaps it is wisest to allow the practice of meditation to unfold naturally so that when we are sincerely inclined we can experience the effects of mantra for ourselves.

MINDFULNESS

When you are resting your attention on the breath or on a mantra you will still be aware of what is passing through your mind. Sometimes the experience is tranquil; at other times thoughts and images may lift your mind on crests of excitement, lower it into troughs of lethargy, toss it about in storms of emotion, and turn it first toward one desire, and then another—it can be difficult to maintain any sort of stability. Throughout your meditation, mindfulness, the natural companion to concentration, can help you.

An Indian village woman whose task in the morning is to go to the well for water practices mindfulness, though she may not know it. As she fills her vessel, balances it on her head, and returns to her home, she is simultaneously talking with friends, wending her way among the stones and exposed roots of the trail, and thinking about her duties for the day. She encounters and manages all the distractions that come before her, but at the same time she maintains her focus without spilling a drop of water.

Mindfulness is a refinement of awareness. When we are mindful we are aware of the mind in its entirety: we see both the focus of attention and the distractions that arise in seeming competition with that focus. The focus is maintained; the distractions are allowed to come and go. Mindfulness permits us to have no reaction—to simply observe the content of the mind and let it pass. We are traveling through, not into, the mind.

In its early stages mindfulness is not so much a state of being as it is a collection of skills that can be learned and practiced. Here are some of them:

- ▶ Recognizing the critical, judgmental self-talks that we apply to our thoughts and feelings, and setting them aside.
- ▶ Witnessing the thoughts and emotions that pass through the mind instead of identifying with them.
- ▶ Becoming one with the thoughts, and thus accepting ourselves as we are.
- ▶ Remaining flexible in the face of the wide variety of thoughts and feelings that demand action or attention.
- ▶ Sensing the depth of emotion that has prompted a given thought, and working with that emotional energy sensitively and patiently.
- ▶ Remaining in the present rather than journeying to the past or future.
- ▶ Recognizing and maintaining the focus of concentration, knowing that this focus is the antidote to being caught up by the train of thought.

Ultimately the combination of mindfulness and concentration evolves into the deeply penetrating state of meditation—an experience that relieves mental pain and nurtures non-attachment. It is an experience focused in the present moment, and it is free of expectations. During this phase of practice the effort to concentrate is fully relaxed. Replacing our conscious effort, the meditative focus now seems to draw us naturally inward toward a stillness that rests our emotions, clears our thinking, awakens our intuition, and provides a sense of abiding peace. This experience is intrinsic to our nature, and with practice we can return to it whenever we choose.

An Outline of Practice

Here is a summary of all the steps in the relaxation/ meditation process.

▶ **Develop a still and steady posture** (lying down for relaxation; sitting for meditation).

▶ **Bring the flow of breath** into your awareness. Don't concern yourself with mechanics at first—just soften your lower ribs and abdomen, and feel the cleansing and nourishing movements of the breath again and again. Then allow the breath to become diaphragmatic.

▶ **Shape the breath.** Let it be deep, smooth, even, without sound, without pause. Let it flow without effort.

▶ **Relax your body** from head to toes, and toes to head, breathing and releasing tension. Then breathe as if the whole body breathes.

▶ In a sitting posture, **focus on the touch of breath** in the nostrils. Be patient as you gradually narrow your attention, detaching from passing thoughts.

▶ **Deepen and lengthen the time** spent with your focus on the breath. Do not condemn distracting thoughts; let them be.

▶ **Relax your mind further** and merge the sound of the breath—the mantra *soham*— with the touch of the breath. Let the sound of the mantra flow effortlessly at the natural pace of your breathing.

▶ **Center your awareness** in the sound where it arises in your mind, with only the merest awareness of the breath.

▶ **Rest in the mantra** and in the center of your being, allowing waves of energy and thought to come and go. The waves are circling around the center, but they are not at the center. You are a relaxed, inner witness, dwelling in the presence of your own being.

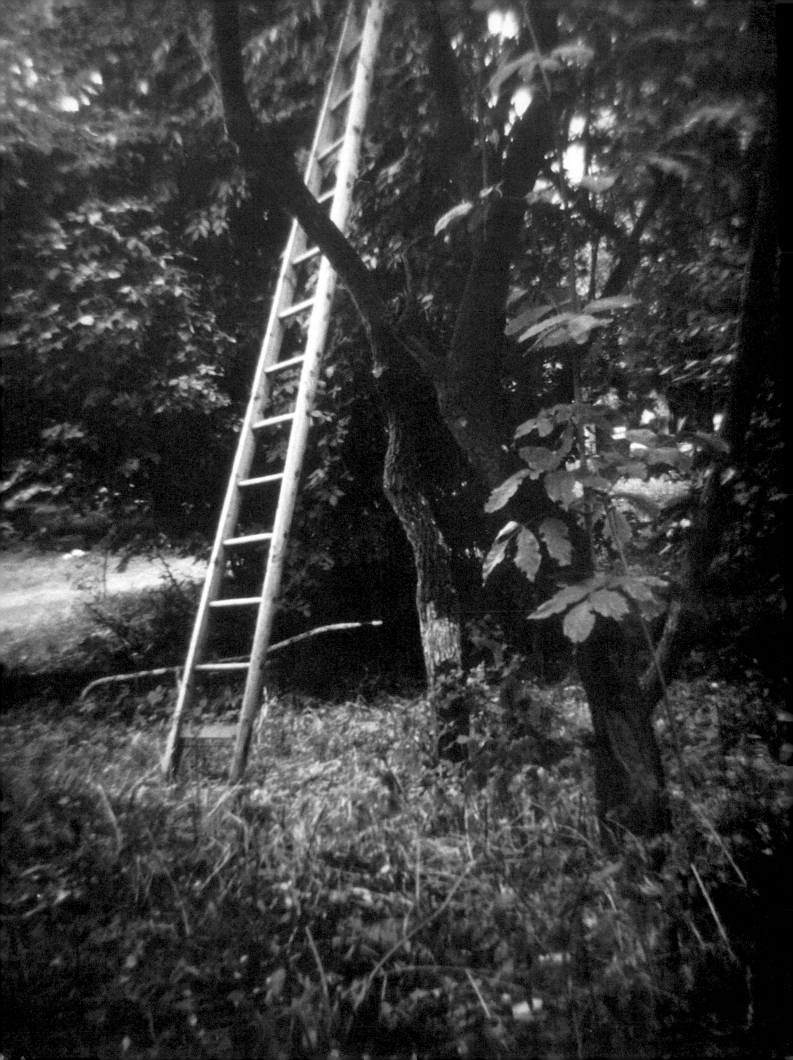

CHAPTER TEN

YOGA IN ACTION

Yoga is skill in action.
—— *Bhagavad Gita*

BREATHING, relaxation, and asana practice, together with sitting for meditation every day, will go a long way toward creating a balanced, cheerful mind, but there are still times when we find ourselves out of sorts. Most of us have developed entrenched habits of living and thinking that undermine our yoga practice—habits that sabotage our peace of mind, compel us to take action we don't really want to take, and divert us from what is most important.

From where do these problems arise, and what does yoga tell us about how to live wisely? To answer, we must first understand that we do not function indepen- dently of our environment. We need food, sunlight, water, shelter, and a secure, comfortable place to sleep. The quality of our energy depends on the quality of these externals; we cannot separate ourselves from them, try as we might. We can, however, choose to invigorate ourselves by acting in harmony with these needs instead of depleting ourselves by going against the flow.

But often we are not aware that we are squandering our energy, nor do we know how to alter our behavior when we realize that we should. We need reliable strate- gies for understanding our relationship with the world and for improving that relationship when necessary.

THE FOUR INSTINCTIVE URGES

Yoga tells us that most of life's problems arise from the way in which we manage four instinctive urges: the desire for food, sleep, sex, and self-preservation. These primitive drives prompt us to perform most of our actions. They are also a primary source of our emotional life, for when our desires are satisfied we are happy (at least momentarily), but when they are thwarted, anger, anxiety, jealousy, and other negative emotions come forward. This dance between desires and emotions is subtle and takes countless forms, but it rarely brings us closer to a sense of inner fulfillment. A desire, once fulfilled, quickly spawns another.

It is obvious that our primal urges can create problems for us. But if channeled wisely these same urges can fuel our creative and compassionate endeavors, as well as inspire our spiritual goals. The secret is awareness— acknowledging the importance of these instincts and discovering how to work with them. To live a balanced life, the yogis say, the four urges need to be wisely regulated. Let's take a brief look at each of them.

FOOD

Once there was a renunciate saint whose mind and body had been rendered pure and sensitive by the long, sustained practice of yoga. Yet one day, after dining with the king, he was suddenly overcome by avarice. Noticing the queen's gem-studded necklace lying on a nearby table, he took it. The next morning, after cleansing his digestive system in the course of his morning ablutions, he remembered what he had done. Shocked, he returned the necklace immediately. Then, determined to discover the cause of his strange behavior, he sat down to reflect,

For one who is moderate in food and pleasure, whose actions are disciplined, whose sleep and waking are balanced, yoga destroys all sorrow.

—*Bhagavad Gita 6:17*

and this prompted him to investigate the source of the food served at the king's table. When he did, he discovered that the grain served that day had been grown, harvested, and marketed by fearful and greedy people. He saw that his mind had been perverted by eating that grain—under its influence he had acquired the same habits that motivated its suppliers.

This story may seem implausible from our modern point of view, but in the yogic view, food has properties that extend beyond its chemical makeup. It influences our physical, mental, emotional, and spiritual life as well. In other words, we take on the subtle characteristics of the food we eat.

Food affects consciousness by first affecting the balance of energy in the body. Stale or heavily processed food has lost its vitality, and eating it leads to a state of dullness and lethargy. Foods that are agitating and overstimulating (such as coffee, sugar, and highly spiced foods) foster angry, impatient, anxious, and fearful mental states. On the other hand, most fresh vegetables, fruits, grains, and legumes, as well as dairy products that are not overly processed, are neither depressing nor stimulating. They nourish and energize, leaving us calm, clear, and content. They increase the qualities of mind and health that we are cultivating in our yogic lifestyle. It follows, then, that by carefully combining and skillfully preparing our food we can increase the overall quality of our diet and thus our lives.

Even perfect food is of no value, however, if we are not able to digest and assimilate it. We may have little choice in how our food is grown, marketed, or cooked, but we can choose how we eat. A number of simple observances will have a positive influence over how our food affects us.

Among these, eating in proportion to our hunger is the most important. Overeating is like smothering a fire by stacking on too much wood. It creates an internal crisis— all our energy rushes to cope with the overload and we either fall asleep or feel dull, lethargic, and polluted.

How to Improve Digestion

► Relax briefly before and after meals.
► Chew thoroughly.
► Eat regular meals.
► Avoid big meals before bed.
► Don't overeat.
► Avoid consuming sugar and caffeine with meals or around mealtime.
► Enjoy your food!

Similarly, snacking throughout the day gives the digestive system no chance to rest. This is also true of eating late at night. Digestion is most efficient when meals are regular and the largest meal is eaten around noon, the time when the digestive fire burns brightest.

Eating on the run, or when angry, upset, or worried, interferes with digestion. In the first place the parasympathetic nervous system (which promotes digestion) functions best when we are calm and receptive; it functions poorly when we are stressed. What is more, when we eat in a hurry we are unable to bring full awareness to the process and thus we deprive ourselves of nourishment at deeper, more subtle levels.

Food sustains life. Eating calmly, with full awareness and gratitude, nurtures the mind and spirit as well as the body; this connects us both with the external world and with our own inner nature. So take a moment before you eat to quietly give thanks for your food, remembering its source and purpose so that it may be integrated into the whole of your life. Then fully enjoy the flavors, colors, and textures of your meal.

How to Improve Your Diet

► Keep a log of what you eat and when.
► Reduce or eliminate snacking.
► Reduce your intake of fat, sugar, and meat.
► Eat calmly, thankfully, and with awareness.
► Make dietary changes gradually.

These suggestions are not ironclad, however, and you will need to experiment to see what works best for you. Don't torture yourself while you move toward more wholesome food choices. As you become more serene and energetic with the practice of yoga, you will naturally gravitate toward a diet that supports that state—a diet based on the deepest needs of the body and mind, not on tastes dictated by the tongue alone.

SLEEP

The four urges are interrelated, so when one is mismanaged it affects the others. If you are eating stale food, for example, you will need more rest than if your food is fresh. Although stale food may contain enough nutrients to sustain life, it has little of the vitality of a peach plucked ripe off the tree, or a tomato fresh from the garden. In other words, when you are feeling tired it may be this vitality you are deprived of, not sleep.

Sleep is itself part of a bigger picture—its quality is affected by the same conditions that disturb us when we are awake, but when we are asleep they affect us at a more subtle level. That is why we can sometimes sleep for hours and still not feel fully rested. Changing our diet, practicing asanas, pranayama, and meditation, and managing our emotions and relationships more successfully will improve the quality of our sleep and reduce the amount we need, thus reversing the trend toward exhaustion.

So will changing our sleep habits. For example, experiment with going to bed on time and getting up on time, and see if the quality of your sleep improves. Living in a climate-controlled, artificially lighted world, we tend to forget that we are connected energetically to the rhythms of the seasons and the days, and that we function much more efficiently if we are on a regular schedule. A routine life (though not a rigid one) has the power to promote good health, renew our energy, focus our attention, and fuel our creativity.

Cultivate a peaceful nervous system and mind before going to bed, and avoid activities that are agitating or disturbing, including strenuous exercise (gentle stretches are good if you're tense or have a lot of nervous energy). Let the time before bed be one of quiet reflection, relaxation, or meditation. Take a warm bath. Find something in the day to be grateful for and something to look forward to on the morrow.

If you have trouble falling asleep, consider cutting down on your intake of caffeine, especially late in the day. A cup of coffee after lunch may keep you awake at bedtime, or even wake you up in the middle of the night—still tired and unable to fall back asleep. And this will prompt you to start the next day with a caffeine boost.

As your yoga practice develops you may find that you need less sleep and want to get up earlier in the morning. As with any habit, a gradual change is much more likely to meet with success than an abrupt one, so begin by getting up 15 minutes earlier than usual every day for a week or two and see how you feel. When you are ready, push your wake-up time back another 15 minutes. In this way you can add a refreshing half hour to your day with relative ease. Try to wake up by setting your intention in your mind before you go to sleep. Otherwise, use a pleasant alarm, not one that startles.

A Sleep Experiment

Going to bed at the right time is energizing, while staying up even a half hour past our optimal bedtime can sap our energy the next day. A simple experiment will illustrate how your sleep schedule affects the way you feel and think. It will also make you aware of your current habits.

To begin, ask yourself, "What is the best time for me to go to bed?" Make a note of it: _____ and then record your actual bedtime for a week. (That means when you get into bed, turn off the lights, and settle in to sleep.) Each day, rate the quality of your sleep and your energy on a scale of 1–10. Note any trends at the end of the week.

Day	Bedtime	Quality of Sleep (1–10)	Energy the Next Day (1–10)

It is difficult to make sudden changes in something as well-rehearsed as sleep habits, so do it gradually. Chances are you will find that going to bed at your best time yields big benefits.

Having Trouble Falling Asleep?

This elegant little technique will put you to sleep and help you sleep more peacefully. It uses an effortless 2-to-1 breath—exhaling about twice as long as you inhale. Observe your breath attentively. Breathe without pauses, jerks, or shakiness. Get into bed and take:

8 breaths lying on your back;
16 breaths lying on your right side;
32 breaths lying on your left side.
Sweet dreams!

—from "Taming the Roller Coaster,"
Yoga International *magazine*

DESIRES

Woven into the fabric of life are two other powerful drives: the urge for sex (and other sensual pleasures), and the urge for self-preservation. Here (as with food and sleep), yoga takes a middle-of-the-road approach. Rigidly controlling or suppressing one of the primitive urges has the effect of disturbing another—for example, depriving yourself of sleep may cause your eating habits to spin out of control. On the other hand, the four primitive drives should not be indulged as if they were the main reason for living.

The true measure of any sensual experience is its effect on thoughts, emotions, moods, and energy. In order to manage the drive for sensual pleasure it is best to create an atmosphere of moderation. Then enjoyment of the senses does not lead either to compulsiveness or to dependence. When pleasure can be experienced without guilt or agitation, and if it does not preoccupy us, then it does not disturb our equilibrium. But if the mind is distracted by an enjoyable experience, then the cause of that disturbance may need to be identified through careful self-observation and addressed through self-discipline.

Cultivating an attitude of contentment is the key to managing our desires, because happiness, according to the sages, is the result not of getting what we want but of feeling content with what we have, unencumbered by hankerings and expectations. With this mind-set we can choose to rest our senses from time to time. This is the idea behind, for example, voluntary periods of juice fasting, observing silence, or abstaining from sex. Such practices not only rejuvenate both body and mind, they also give us opportunities for deepening spiritual awareness.

SELF-PRESERVATION

The urge for self-preservation is deeply embedded in everyone, and when danger threatens it is quickly activated. It blossoms in the form of fear, anxiety, and anger—powerful emotions that can mobilize tremendous amounts of energy. Unfortunately, however, in daily affairs these reactions are often out of proportion to the dangers we actually encounter, and the levels of apprehension and anger we sustain burden our body and mind.

We usually equate self-preservation with the basic survival instinct, but it has a more subtle dimension as well. Each of us is attached to many things that are not essential to our survival but are precious to us nonetheless, and through these attachments we create numberless identities. For example, the placement of our seat at a wedding banquet may signify our social status; our collection of jazz recordings may be the last remnants of pride in a childhood musical talent; a newly purchased car may symbolize our financial ranking. When these identities (or the objects that represent them) are endangered, it triggers the urge for self-preservation—sometimes as if our very life were being threatened. And the more rigidly we are attached to these identities, the more overreactive our emotional alarm system.

Managing the urge for self-preservation requires wisdom and discrimination. In yoga we are never asked to violate our common sense or to disregard appropriate fears and concerns, and we certainly do not need to give up our possessions and social standing to remain inwardly balanced. Instead, we can soften the rigidity of our attachments so that they do not create problems for us. We can learn to moderate our reactions, recognizing and sorting out essentials from non-essentials. Without such flexibility, fear and anger will disturb our health and peace of mind and move us further from our goal.

TEN PRINCIPLES OF SELF-REGULATION

We know that if the four primitive urges are not wisely regulated they lead to self-defeating habits that are difficult to overcome. The yoga tradition offers a way to change unproductive habit patterns through a set of ten powerful guidelines for everyday living: the *yamas* (restraints) and *niyamas* (observances), the first two rungs of the ladder of raja yoga. The yamas and niyamas show us how to manage our relationships with ourselves, with others, and with the world around us. Through them, we can transform ourselves and bring our spiritual goals into daily life.

The Restraints	*Yamas*
non-harming	ahimsa
truthfulness	satya
non-stealing	asteya
moderation of the senses	brahmacharya
non-possessiveness	aparigraha

The Observances	*Niyamas*
self-purification	shaucha
contentment	santosha
self-discipline	tapas
self-study	svadhyaya
self-surrender	Ishvara pranidhana

The five yamas (the restraints) stop the drain of energy that takes place when we become lost in the four primitive urges. They alert us when our current actions are out of sync with our spiritual aspirations, and they prompt us to restrain unproductive behaviors and replace them with new and more productive ones. By practicing the yamas we learn to understand the psychological processes behind our actions, and as a result we become more skillful at managing emotional disturbances.

The five niyamas (the observances) are constructive tools for cultivating happiness and self-confidence; the opportunities to practice them arise wherever you may find yourself. If the yamas are like the banks of a river, restraining the haphazard flow of inner energies, then the niyamas are the disciplines and observances that propel this stream forward toward its goal.

THE FIVE RESTRAINTS (YAMAS)
Non-Harming (Ahimsa)

In Sanskrit the prefix *a* means "not," while *himsa* means "harming, injuring, killing, or doing violence." *Ahimsa*, the first of the yamas and the highest-ranking among them, is the practice of non-harming or non-violence. This is the key, the sages tell us, to maintaining both harmonious relationships in the world and a tranquil inner life.

Ahimsa arises through awareness, the same skill we have practiced in asanas and meditation. By observing ourselves in terms of ahimsa we can see the almost invariable spiral of fear, anger, and blame that precedes aggressive actions, and we can notice how violence often results from projecting our own pain onto our surroundings. With practice, awareness of these inner cues alerts us when something is wrong, and then we can stop ourselves from reacting with automatic hostility.

At a deeper level, ahimsa is less a conscious process than a natural consequence of yoga practice. As our journey unfolds it leads to awareness of the peaceful and enduring core that is our true nature; the desire to prevent harm is a spontaneous expression of that awareness. We begin to realize that the inner self in others is identical to our own inner self, and we wish no harm to come to any being.

But the practice of ahimsa that often proves most challenging is applying the principle of non-harming to ourselves. Self-criticism, self-doubt, and the inability to forgive our past mistakes take a heavy toll; they undermine our confidence and our will. And once we have lost our equilibrium, then fear, anger, and guilt leave us vulnerable to further negative thoughts.

The principle of non-harming reverses this process. It shows us how to love ourselves and others, and when ahimsa is fully embraced an inner confidence emerges that is deep-seated and surprisingly powerful. Great teachers of every age have maintained that through practicing non-violence we can transform ourselves and our universe. For example, the first precept attributed to the early Greek physician Hippocrates, the father of modern medicine, was "Do no harm."

It is true that ahimsa admonishes us to maintain inner control, but it does not restrict us from acting assertively when necessary. If anything, once we have committed ourselves to non-violence we will begin to search more actively for ways to handle conflict, prevent pain, and fulfill our needs. But this is a process that unfolds over time; as the experience of non-harming becomes integrated into daily life it works its own magic on us and on those around us.

Truthfulness (Satya)

The word *sat,* in Sanskrit, means "that which exists, that which is." *Satya,* in turn, means "truthfulness"—seeing and reporting things as they are rather than the way we would like them to be. When we are truthful life is uncomplicated and well-anchored, but when we attempt to conceal or modify reality our motives are suspect, and our confidence in ourselves and one another is undermined.

Satya is a challenge to the heart as well as the intellect. Most often when we are tempted to speak or act untruthfully it is because we fear that being truthful will create conflict in our lives or prevent us from obtaining what we desire. So to avoid such pain we usually do not tell out-and-out lies—we simply distort things a bit. We gain what we want through partial truths that seem quite easy to justify, and a pattern of self-deceit develops that is very difficult to reverse. The goal of satya is to prevent us from becoming more and more entangled in this web and losing the ability to observe our thoughts and feelings dispassionately.

As with all the yamas, the task of practicing truthfulness leads us in two directions. Inwardly we learn to recognize the cascade of fears and other negative emotions that prompt us to twist reality. Then, once we have understood and processed these fears, our thoughts, speech, and actions can be realigned with the truth, and we can look more deeply into our needs and desires. Outwardly, in the practice of satya, we refrain from telling lies.

When we are relating to others, however, being truthful is not an excuse to blurt out what we may really be thinking. Truthfulness does not replace tact and discrimination—remember, we are also practicing non-harming. Satya means being aware that speaking the truth can be hurtful, and then speaking with kindness and compassion as well as clarity. It means looking for the positive, and being tactful about the negative. In other words, when it is necessary to speak unpleasant truths, we do it without the intention to hurt, and we speak as skillfully as possible.

In the end, truthfulness preserves inner order. Through it we remain well-grounded in our relationships with others as well as within ourselves. And the stability spawned from this leads naturally to more lofty truths, ones with the power to inspire us in our search for inner peace.

Non-Stealing (Asteya)

The word *steya* means "stealing." When it is combined with the prefix *a* it is negated, yielding *asteya:* non-stealing. This is the third yama, the prohibition against taking for ourselves what belongs to another. We are most likely to associate stealing with tangible objects, but intangibles such as information and emotional favors are more likely to be the objects stolen in our world. And even though most of us do not knowingly or habitually steal, it is sometimes not so far from our minds as we would like to imagine.

The urge to steal arises from a sense of unhappiness, incompleteness, and envy. It thrives on the belief that we have been unjustly deprived, and on the fear that we will not get what we want. Anger is often used to justify the impulse to steal, and secrecy is its constant ally. As in many other situations in which we spend our energy unwisely and consequently lose self-esteem, our own sense of emptiness is the ultimate robber here. The psychological process leading to stealing is like pouring milk into a bowl with a hole in the bottom—no matter how much is poured in, the bowl always remains empty. Our emotional needs are not met by possessing what we know is not ours.

The prescription is to plug the hole in the bowl. Whenever the thought of gaining something illicitly arises, set it aside at once. Do not give a second thought to what may come to you outside of legitimate channels. Depend entirely on the resources of your own life for your happiness. You will immediately find your mind freed of guilt and filled with quiet confidence.

But if the practice of asteya is a problem for you, the solution is to give. We rarely recall what we have taken with any satisfaction, but we remember with joy how it feels to have given. So give food; give money; give time. Practice giving any chance you get. Since wealth is ultimately a state of mind, you will feel increasingly wealthy. In fact, so long as you are selfless in your giving, the great yogic texts say that your sense of inner wealth will bring you outer wealth.

Moderating the Senses (Brahmacharya)

The literal translation of *brahmacharya* is "walking in God-consciousness." Practically speaking, this means that brahmacharya turns the mind inward, balancing and supervising the senses, and leads to freedom from dependencies and cravings. And yogis tell us that when the mind is freed from domination by the senses, sensual pleasures are replaced by inner joy.

The problem, however, is that the same mind that is accustomed to banqueting on sensual experiences is also being asked to regulate itself. As a consequence, it can easily justify opening the doors to sensual pleasures but struggles to find even a few reasons for closing them again.

Brahmacharya offers a practical strategy for handling this dilemma, one that simply and elegantly addresses one of life's most difficult problems: when the senses are awake and active, it counsels, watch them—allow them moderate activity, and then stop them. This is not so much constraining the senses as it is giving the mind a chance to shift away from their distractions. It takes diligence to remember this in the midst of an ice cream feast or an encounter with chocolate, yet the principle is surprisingly effective: Enjoy in moderation. When your mind tells you that you are acting immoderately—stop.

But what is moderation? Sometimes the mind is so befuddled by the senses that it has lost all sense of proportion. The trick is to remember that both overindulgence and repression deplete our vital force. Both leave us insecure and anxious, and it becomes difficult to gather our energies again. So when sense pleasures seem to be weakening or mis-channeling our energy, they need further attention.

Brahmacharya practices range from the very structured to the highly intuitive. A person who craves candy bars may need to impose a limit of one per day, while a person who rarely eats candy bars can go ahead and have one when the urge arises. Making wise choices about the books and magazines we read, the movies we see, and the company we keep will help us conserve energy and keep our mind focused and dynamic. Being moderate in all sensual activities so that we don't dwell on them, staying committed and faithful to one partner in a relationship that is mutually supportive—this is the middle path of brahmacharya.

Non-Possessiveness (Aparigraha)

Graha means "to grasp" and *pari* means "things": *aparigraha* means "not grasping things," or non-possessiveness. It helps us achieve a balanced relationship with the things that we each call "mine."

Our relationship with an object in the world changes when we become its owner. The transition is subtle, but it is easy to tell if the process has gone haywire. Here are some unmistakable signs: we take better care of an object in our possession than one belonging to someone else; we are unwilling to share what we already have enough of; we acquire more of something than we can use; the sheer number of our possessions encumbers us. In other words, when we over-identify with our possessions—obtaining them, holding on to them, or mourning their loss—then we need aparigraha.

There is a yogic maxim that makes the point clear. "All the things of the world," it says, "are yours to use, but not to own." That is the essence of aparigraha. Whenever we become possessive, we are in turn possessed, anxiously holding onto our things and grasping for more. On the other hand, when we make good use of the possessions that come to us and enjoy them without becoming emotionally dependent on them, then they neither wield power over us nor lead to false identities and expectations.

Ultimately, aparigraha extends to interpersonal relationships. When we depend too much on others, give more in a relationship than is healthy for us, replace mutual give-and-take with the need for tightfisted control, or attempt to increase our self-esteem by gaining someone else's love, then we reveal flaws in our underlying perspectives. The practice of non-possessiveness helps us to examine our assumptions and guides us back to the knowledge that even though we cannot own other people, we can establish healthy and productive relationships with them.

THE FIVE OBSERVANCES (NIYAMAS)
Self-Purification (Shaucha)

Shaucha means "purification; cleanliness." It includes a number of techniques for cleansing the body as well as the mind, and it has even been called the aim of the entire system of yoga. Why does it have such significance? The sages say that shaucha is not only the foundation for bodily health, it is also the doorway to deeper and more tranquil states of meditation.

Connections between purification and health are easy to identify. For example, the dramatic lengthening of the

human lifespan over the past century is widely attributed to improvements in sanitation. And the need for cleanliness both when handling food and in medical situations is well-established. But purification has an even more intimate relationship with our health. The body, breath, and mind are all undergoing constant change—old cells are replaced by new ones, the breath ebbs and flows; thoughts enter and depart in a seemingly endless procession. At every layer of our being nutrients are continually taken in and wastes discharged.

Blockages in the flow at any level are an invitation to trouble. And from the yogic point of view the accumulation of internal wastes (whether in the form of undigested food or undigested experience) is the primary cause of disease. The aim of shaucha is to remove internal toxins and wastes, and to select wisely from the many choices of food, emotions, and thoughts waiting to come in.

When the body is purified it enjoys physical health; when the mind is purified it becomes increasingly clear, friendly, and cheerful. It does not hold on to fear or anger, and self-doubts vanish quickly. All of these benefits, both internal and external, come about through the practice of yoga.

It is not difficult to recognize moments in life when shaucha can be applied productively. The trick is to grasp those moments and use them. For as the texts say, once the heart is purified, then the mind becomes one-pointed; when the mind is centered, the senses become calm; and when the senses are calmed, the way to self-realization is prepared.

Contentment (Santosha)

The word santosha means "contentment" as well as "delight, happiness, joy." We tend to equate it with the satisfaction of desires, but yogis tell us that true contentment is something quite different. The happiness which arises from fulfilling desires, they point out, is soon clouded by the birth of more cravings and frustrations. Contentment, they say, is quite different. It unfolds from an experience of acceptance—of life, of ourselves, and of whatever life has brought to us. Contentment is an aspect of living in the moment. When we are content, we are happy. Thus—and here is the key to this niyama— through the power of contentment, happiness becomes our choice.

But how do we achieve contentment when inwardly we are disappointed and striving for change and improvement? The answer is actually more practical than we might imagine: We create it. We commit ourselves to the yogic premise that whatever we have in the present moment is enough. And once we do this, happiness will find an enduring place in our lives; whatever aspirations we have for the future will simply add to our joy.

Practicing contentment means letting go of the past. It means not condemning ourselves for not being wiser, wealthier, or more successful than we are. It also means that we must free our mind of expectations. Then we will see life in a larger context and be able to ride its ups and downs with equanimity. Contentment allows us to know that we are making the right effort. Contentment also leads us to the next niyama, tapas, which complements and completes it.

Self-Discipline (Tapas)

The literal definition of *tapas* is "heat," in this case the heat that builds during periods of determined effort. Tapas accompanies any discipline that is willingly and gladly accepted in order to bring about a change of some kind—whether it be improved health, a new habit, better concentration, or a different direction in life. Tapas focuses energy, creates fervor, and increases strength and confidence. The practice of asanas is a form of tapas for the body; meditation is a tapas that purifies and focuses the mind.

But tapas is not so much a specific action as it is the concerted internal effort that accompanies the action. Tapas can go hand in hand with any task—even something as mundane as cleaning the bathroom floor. Whenever we perform our actions with full determination and effort, they are performed with tapas. Just as a light beam can be focused and reorganized into a powerful laser, so does our determination focus diverse energies to increase internal fire. Far from the mindlessness of heavy-handed discipline, true tapas generates ardor and enthusiasm.

What is the value of performing actions with conscious determination and self-discipline? Picture a pile of stacked wood being gradually consumed by a steady flame. The fire both purifies and transforms— impurities are turned to ash while the energy contained in the wood is liberated in the form of light and heat. Acts of tapas are similar. They reduce lethargy, sloth, discouragement, doubt, and the ill-effects of past actions to ashes; they liberate energy in the form of light and heat—in our case, joy and productive action.

A word of practical advice about tapas: be realistic. Through the ardor of tapas we may choose to make healthy changes in our life, but focusing on only one or two changes at a time is usually the best course. Take small steps that can be accomplished successfully. Find replacements for habits that are unproductive. And finally, if you find yourself focused on failure, remember that guilt magnifies its negative effects and keeps you preoccupied with the event that generated it in the first place. Forgive yourself easily while redoubling your determination and self-discipline.

Self-Study (Svadhyaya)

Svadhyaya means, literally, "to recollect (to remember, to contemplate, to meditate on) the self." It is the effort to know the self that shines as the innermost core of our being. By now, however, it must be apparent that within the context of yoga the word "self" requires some careful handling. In the everyday sense "study of the self" implies self-analysis—the effort to gain a clearer understanding of our personality. Yoga approaches the theme of self-study quite differently. It acknowledges that analysis can provide important information, but yogis have long believed that no matter how many hours we give to it, self-analysis will not free us from the tensions of everyday existence. For that we must dive deeper.

Self-study begins with the study of writings that inspire us to feel the presence of the indwelling spirit. They encourage us by illustrating how life is transformed when we learn to concentrate and rest within. For example, this is how the *Bhagavad Gita* describes the joy of self-awareness: "One whose joy is within, who finds contentment within, whose light is within—such a yogi attains the enduring bliss of the self." (5:24)

But inspiring as it is, such knowledge is of little use if we cannot apply it to ourselves. In the second stage of self-study we gain a working knowledge of ourselves through practicing the yamas and niyamas, the asanas, breath awareness, and meditation, and we learn to recognize when we are acting in harmony with our goals and when we are unconsciously acting counter to them. At this stage self-awareness, contemplation, and mindfulness are powerful tools.

Over time, self-study is directed increasingly inward. When mantra is introduced into our meditation practice, it establishes a direct link to the self within. We sense an inward quietude, a state that lingers in our daily life, reducing conflict and calling us back again when our meditation time approaches.

Self-study is not prescriptive. Any practice of yoga can be part of it, as can the words of yogis, saints, and sages, as well as inspiration gained through the teachers we are drawn to. Follow your heart in choosing your path of study, and let it nurture you.

Self-Surrender (Ishvara Pranidhana)

Ishvara refers to all-pervading consciousness; *pranidhana* means "to surrender." Together, these words are most frequently translated as "self-surrender," the last and most important of the niyamas, and perhaps the most difficult for students to embrace. The problem, of course, lies with the word "surrender." To many of us it implies defeat—our will overwhelmed and forced into submission. And what could be more offensive to our sense of independence and self-responsibility than this?

To understand the importance of Ishvara pranidhana let us return briefly to the four instinctive urges: food, sleep, sex, and self-preservation. Appeasing them is an endless job. They can be regulated but never fully satisfied. When the four urges dictate the flow of life the pursuit of happiness inevitably becomes dependent on externals. And one purpose of the yamas and niyamas is to regulate our wants so that life doesn't become an endless round of such cravings and attachments.

Along with the four primitive urges, however, there is another powerful inner drive: the urge for self-realization. As strong and inexhaustible as the other four, this fifth urge is fulfilled through attending to our inner life, and its call is the voice of our inner self. When the outer world distracts us it slips away, only to return later and call again.

Yoga shows us how to answer this call. Through the practical experiences we gather in our quest we are inspired to practice more. Our enthusiasm is tested and strengthened by the demands of daily life. We may make choices that seem illogical to those who do not know about the inner journey we have embraced, but we feel at ease about the direction our life has taken.

Self-surrender, then, is not a process of defeat or of mindlessly submitting to another's will. It is the act of giving ourselves to a higher purpose—and when we do we feel uplifted and invigorated. This may take place in the midst of a decision-making process, or in discovering a point of view that is better than our own, but it occurs most often when we are meditating, when we let go of the thoughts and desires that bind our thinking process and give one-pointed attention to the center of our being. At such times we transcend the limitations of our attachments and sense the presence of inner stillness. In whatever form it presents itself, that experience, the sages tell us, guides us toward wholeness and the fulfillment of our inward quest.

Each of us approaches yoga from a different point of view, and the wide variety of paths and practices to choose from can easily feel overwhelming. You will need to experiment in order to find what is most suitable for you—a path that fits your personality, a well-balanced selection of practices, and a proportioned time commitment.

The collection of yoga disciplines you select and the effort you invest in them is called *sadhana*. For example, you may choose to practice only a few regularly rehearsed techniques, or a highly evolved routine. You may be diligent about reading and further study, or simply happy to find time to attend a weekly class. But as the weeks and months go by and your practice continues uninterruptedly, it becomes your sadhana.

If you were to organize your daily practice, how might it look? In the early morning the mind is receptive, fresh, and impressionable. Whatever you take in then tends to set the tone for the rest of the day. That's why morning is considered the prize time for practice. In the evening, as the energies of the day are quieted, there is another natural time for practice because as night falls the thoughts of the day can be processed and assimilated, and the mind turned toward deeper awareness. But any time can be suitable for yoga, and your schedule may provide you with other opportunities—ones better fitted to you.

Practice what is appealing to you. If, for example, something you have read or heard makes little sense, set it aside until you have gathered more information. Yoga routines change over time, so allow your practice to mature by reading, attending classes, and meeting with others who are interested in yoga. When asked what was the greatest blessing for someone on the path of yoga, the sage Vasishtha replied, "The company of others on the same path."

Attempting to learn too many new practices at once can be as unproductive as investing too little energy. Focus on one or two things at a time—daily relaxation, hatha yoga sessions, pranayama practice, meditation, nourishing meals, or the effort to stay even-tempered in situations that might normally arouse strong emotions. Gradually build these new skills into your lifestyle. And finally, if you have not already compiled a list of your own, here's a selection of practices that includes something for everyone.

EARLY MORNING

▶ Loosen up and clear your mind with a warm shower and a nasal wash.

▶ Do a sequence of stretches and asanas (a videotape or audiotape may help).

▶ Practice relaxation (lying down if you have done your asanas).

▶ Perform selected breathing practices.

▶ Meditate (this can be done before asana practice if you prefer).

▶ Set aside quiet time for contemplation, prayer, or brief reflective reading.

▶ Eat a breakfast of whole foods.

▶ Plan your morning—the time of day that is often the most productive.

MIDMORNING

▶ A good time for a short diaphragmatic breathing break (skip the coffee and donut—try a piece of fruit if you're hungry).

▶ Loosen tense muscles with shoulder rolls, a twist, and a side bend.

MIDDAY

▶ Consider a few stretches or alternate nostril breathing before lunch.

▶ Pause for relaxed breathing or a prayer before eating.

▶ Eat a meal of whole foods that satisfies your physical needs but won't lead to a post-lunch slump.

▶ Walk a bit to help with digestion before getting back to other activities.

MIDAFTERNOON

▶ Check your breathing to make sure it is free and diaphragmatic.

▶ A few spinal twists in your chair can relieve tension.

▶ Plan the rest of the day, remembering that it is often the least productive time for work activities, so use it for routine tasks, to tie up loose ends, and to prepare for the next day.

LATE AFTERNOON

▶ A good time for brisk exercise—a swim, tennis, or a hatha yoga class.

▶ Finish with a breathing exercise and a short relaxation to shed the tensions of the day and prepare for evening.

EARLY EVENING

▶ Select your supper with grains, legumes, and vegetables in mind; finish eating early so that your body can digest the food and prepare for sleep.

▶ Unwind after supper with some gardening, a family activity, or another enjoyable pastime.

BEFORE BEDTIME

▶ Read something inspiring or comforting.

▶ Remember "contentment"—it will help you establish enduring happiness within and without.

▶ Pray, relax, or meditate to shed the distractions of the day, restore your inward awareness, and prepare you for sleep.

INDEX OF POSTURES

in English & Sanskrit

ABOUT THE AUTHORS

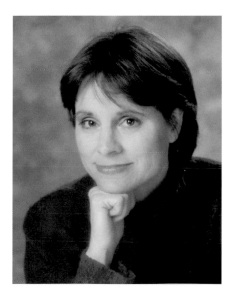

Sandra Anderson is a long-time student of yoga and meditation in the tradition of the Himalayan Institute. A contributing editor of *Yoga International* magazine, she began writing her popular asana column in 1992. She is a Board member of the Himalayan Institute Teachers Association and trains yoga teachers in New York, Chicago, Pittsburgh, and other cities. She administers a Sanskrit correspondence course as well as the Institute's Center for Health and Healing. She has been practicing and teaching yoga since 1981.

Before taking up residency at the Himalayan Institute, Sandra worked throughout the West as an environmental groundwater geologist. She studied geology at the University of Nebraska and the University of New Mexico. She currently lives at the Himalayan Institute's headquarters in Honesdale, Pennsylvania, where she is part of the teaching faculty.

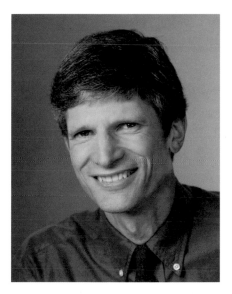

Rolf Sovik, Psy.D., is spiritual director of the Himalayan Institute and co-director (along with his wife, Mary Gail) of the Himalayan Institute of Buffalo, New York. He is also a clinical psychologist in private practice, with a special interest in applying yoga in the treatment and prevention of mental health problems. He has been practicing, teaching, and training teachers within the Himalayan Institute tradition since 1972. He holds a doctorate in psychology from the Minnesota School of Professional Psychology; a master's degree in Eastern studies from the University of Scranton; and an undergraduate degree (magna cum laude) with majors in philosophy (honors) and history from St. Olaf College. He has studied yoga both in the U.S. and in India and Nepal and was initiated as a pandit in the Himalayan tradition in 1987. He is a board member of the Himalayan Institute Teachers Association and a regular contributor to *Yoga International* magazine.

RECOMMENDED BOOKS

SELECTED BOOKS BY SRI SWAMI RAMA

Living With the Himalayan Masters

His expereiences with the great teachers who guided his life.

Meditation and its Practice

Basic tools for starting a meditation practice or deepening an existing one.

Science of Breath

How proper breathing helps physical and mental health and attain higher states of consciousness.

Art of Joyful Living

A simple philosophy of living and practical suggestions for being happy.

SELECTED BOOKS BY PANDIT RAJMANI TIGUNAIT

The Power of Mantra and the Mystery of Initiation

An introduction to the science of mantra and its relation to meditative states.

Inner Quest

Answers to the most frequently asked questions about yoga and spirituality.

At the Eleventh Hour

Much deeper than a sequence of astonishing events in the life of Swami Rama.

Himalayan Masters: A Living Tradition

About eight masters who knew how to live in the world while experiencing the innermost truth.

OTHER BOOKS

Diet and Nutrition and *Transition to Vegetarianism* (Rudolph Ballentine, M.D.)

Comprehensive books on the principles and practice of vegetarian eating.

The Muscle Book and *Stretching Without Pain* (Paul Blakey)

About muscles and how to take care of them.

GUIDED PRACTICE TAPES

Yoga: Mastering the Basics—Flexibility, Strength, and Balance (videocassette)
and *Yoga: Mastering the Basics—Deepening and Strengthening* (videocassette)
   Guided asana practices corresponding to Asana Sequence One and Two
   respectively of this book. (book and both videos can be purchased as a
   set through the Himalayan Institute Press)

* New CD: Gently Guided Relaxations (CD / 60 minutes; Rolf Sovik, Psy.D.)
   Four methods to rest your body, calm your nervous system, and relax the
   mind.
Learn to Meditate and *Guided Relaxation & Breathing* (audiocasettes, Rolf
Sovik, Psy.D.)
   Guided practices of relaxation, meditation and breath training.
Guided Meditation for Beginners (audiocassette/24 minutes; Swami Rama)
   Instruction on the beginning stages of meditation from a renowned
   master, including a brief guided practice.
Joints and Glands Exercises (audiocassette/60 minutes)
   Designed specially for those with limited physical abilities and those
   wishing a more gentle series of stretches and movements.

For a complete catalog or to order Himalayan Institute publications and
products, contact:

Himalayan Institute Press
630 Main Street, Suite 350
Honesdale, PA 18431–1843
800-822-4547 Fax: 570-647-1552
Email: hibooks@HimalayanInstitute.org
Web: www.HimalayanInstitute.org

THE HIMALAYAN INSTITUTE

A leader in the field of yoga, meditation, spirituality, and holistic health, the Himalayan Institute was founded by Swami Rama of the Himalayas. The mission of the Himalayan Institute is Swami Rama's mission—to discover and embrace the sacred link—the spirit of human heritage that unites East and West, spirituality and science, and ancient wisdom and modern technology. Using timetested techniques of yoga, Ayurveda, integrative medicine, principles of spirituality, and holistic health, the Institute has brought health, happiness, peace and prosperity to the lives of tens of thousands for more than a quarter of a century. At the Himalayan Institute you will learn techniques to develop a healthy body, a clear mind, and a joyful spirit, bringing a qualitative change within and without.

The Himalayan Institute's headquarters is located on a beautiful 400-acre campus in the rolling hills of the Pocono Mountains of northeastern Pennsylvania. In the spiritually vibrant atmosphere of the Institute you will meet students and seekers from all walks of life who are participating in programs in hatha yoga, meditation, stress reduction, Ayurveda, nutrition, spirituality, and eastern philosophy. Choose from weekend or weeklong seminars, monthlong self-transformation programs, longer residential programs, spiritual retreats, and custom-designed holistic health services, pancha karma, and rejuvenation programs. In the peaceful setting of the Institute, you will relax and discover the best of yourself. We invite you to join us in the ongoing process of personal growth and development.

Swami Rama transplanted his Himalayan cave to the Poconos in the form of the Himalayan Institute. The wisdom you will find at the Institute will direct you to the safe, secure, peaceful and joyful cave in your own heart.

"Knowledge of various paths leads you to form your own conviction. The more you know, the more you decide to learn."
—Swami Rama

PROGRAMS AND SERVICES INCLUDE:
- ▶ Weekend or extended seminars and workshops
- ▶ Meditation retreats and advanced meditation instruction
- ▶ Hatha yoga teachers training
- ▶ Residential programs for self-development
- ▶ Holistic health services and Pancha Karma at the Institute's Center for Health and Healing
- ▶ Spiritual excursions
- ▶ Varcho Veda® herbal products
- ▶ Himalayan Institute Press
- ▶ *Yoga International* Magazine
- ▶ Correspondence courses

Living Joyfully magazine includes a quarterly guide to programs and is free within the USA. To request a copy, or for further information, call 800-822-4547 or 570-253-5551, write the Himalayan Institute, RR 1 Box 1127, Honesdale, PA 18431-9706 USA, or visit our Web site at www.HimalayanInstitute.org.

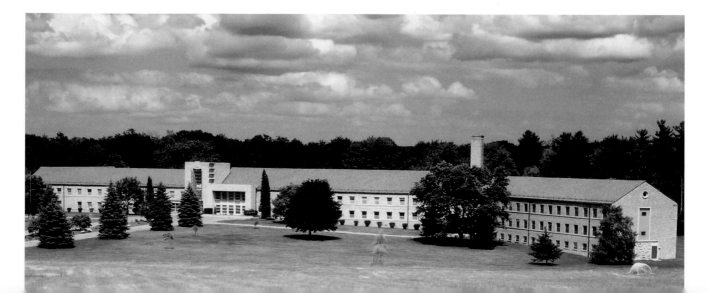

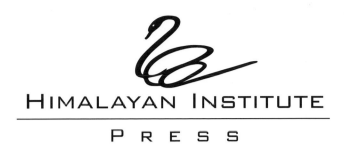

HIMALAYAN INSTITUTE

PRESS

The Himalayan Institute Press has long been regarded as "The Resource for Holistic Living." We publish dozens of titles, as well as audio and video tapes, that offer practical methods for living harmoniously and achieving inner balance. Our approach addresses the whole person—body, mind, and spirit—integrating the latest scientific knowledge with ancient healing and self-development techniques.

We offer a wide array of titles on physical and psychological health and well-being, spiritual growth through meditation and other yogic practices, and translations of yogic scriptures.

Our sidelines include the Japa Kit for meditation practice, the Neti™ Pot, the ideal tool for sinus and allergy sufferers, and The Breath Pillow,™ a unique tool for learning health-supportive diaphragmatic breathing.

Subscriptions are available to a bimonthly magazine, *Yoga International*, which offers thought-provoking articles on all aspects of meditation and yoga, including yoga's sister science, Ayurveda.

For a free catalog:
call 800-822-4547 or 570-253-5551
email hibooks@himalayaninstitute.org
fax 570-647-1552
write Himalayan Institute Press, 630 Main Street, Suite 350,
Honesdale, PA 18431-1843, USA
or visit our Web site at www.himalayaninstitute.org.